Dental, Oral and Maxillofacial Surgery
A Guide to Hospital Practice

Dental, Oral and Maxillofacial Surgery

A Guide to Hospital Practice

Dental, Oral and Maxillofacial Surgery

A Guide to Hospital Practice

DAVID POSWILLO
DDS, MDhc, DSc, FDS, FRACDS, Hon FFD, FIBiol, FRCPath
Professor of Oral and Maxillofacial Surgery, United Medical and Dental Schools of Guy's and St Thomas's Hospitals, University of London

ALEX BABAJEWS
MB, BS, BDS, FDS, FFD, FRCS(Ed)
Senior Registrar, Oral and Maxillofacial Surgery, Royal Surrey County Hospital, Guildford

MALCOLM BAILEY
MB, BS, BDS, FDS, FRCS(Ed)
Consultant Oral and Maxillofacial Surgeon, Queen Mary's Hospital, Roehampton, London and Ashford Hospital, Middlesex

MURRAY FOSTER
MB, BCh, BDS, MScD, FFD, FDS, FRCS(Ed)
Consultant Oral and Maxillofacial Surgeon, North Manchester, Tameside and Oldham General Hospitals

WILLIAM HEINEMANN MEDICAL BOOKS
LONDON

First published in 1986
by William Heinemann Medical Books
22 Bedford Square
London WC1B 3HH

ISBN 0 433 25641 9

Typeset by Wilmaset, Birkenhead, Wirral
Printed in Great Britain by
Redwood Burn Ltd., Trowbridge, Wiltshire

Contents

Foreword

There has long been a need for a pocket manual which will assist the senior dental student or house officer to find, at short notice, those procedures which should be commenced for a patient in need of specialist treatment in the dental, oral and maxillofacial unit.

There have been, in the past, numerous handbooks on both sides of the Atlantic, designed to meet this need in general surgery and medicine, and some other specialised areas. It is refreshing, therefore, to find a book produced by British colleagues which will meet this important need for trainees in our own speciality.

David Poswillo and his co-authors (all of whom have previously worked with him as senior registrars during their training) have had considerable practical experience of hospital oral surgery. They have seen the problems of practice from the viewpoint of trainees, consultants and teachers. Here, they bring together the essentials of present day diagnostic, therapeutic and management principles in a clear, instructive manner, to enable the newly initiated to deal effectively with dental, oral and maxillofacial problems.

I have long deplored the fragmentation of the dental profession into small esoteric specialities, but with the ever widening spectrum in the field of oral and maxillofacial surgery, particularly in orthognathic surgery, a sound dental training is essential for a successful operative procedure.

Therefore I congratulate the authors on refraining from further splitting dental practice into oral and maxillofacial surgery, as I believe that a knowledge of the difficulties and complications of all aspects of surgical endeavour in the region of the mouth and jaws should be essential for the general dental surgeon and trainee specialist alike.

So it is with great pleasure that I commend this work to all dental surgeons who first see these patients, and to those young people into whose hands these cases eventually come.

Sir Terence Ward CBE, 1986

Foreword

Preface

The principles of dental, oral and maxillofacial surgery are taught in the modern undergraduate curriculum. The surgical experience necessary to perform, expeditiously, the clinical procedures involved can only be acquired by practice; many believe that this is best obtained by appointment to suitable posts in the hospital sector soon after graduation.

There are available today excellent textbooks on oral diagnosis and treatment planning and the principles of management of orofacial disease. Several of these are listed in the bibliography at the end of this guide. However, there has long been the need for a pocketbook which will summarise, in brief notes, the myriad things that the senior student or newly appointed house officer must learn, in quick succession, if clinical training is to proceed smoothly with maximum benefit to their patients.

This work is designed mainly to meet that need. In no sense should this small compendium be considered a textbook for those who have completed training in the ever-expanding speciality. In a book of this size much of the finer detail must be omitted. However, it is hoped that the material included will also provide a rapid review of the subject for those who seek an update on the speciality, especially those taking higher examinations which may include questions, written, oral or practical, of a surgical nature.

Different clinicians may vary in the way they proceed with their examination and treatment. There is, however, sufficient common ground in a dental surgical specialty to warrant a general guide such as this. It is the authors' hope that this Guide to Practice will help to standardise various aspects of investigation and management and present a practical answer to those puzzling problems which crowd in on all who, of necessity, receive their initiation by fire. It is their conviction that knowing where to look for the answer is the quickest and safest route to solving a problem!

D. Poswillo, A. Babajews, M. Bailey, M. Foster, 1986

Preface

Acknowledgements

We thank Jean Perry for help with the illustrations, and all our secretaries who struggled to produce the typed drafts. We are most grateful to Dr A.L. Gwynne of The Medical Defence Union who contributed our section on record keeping, and to Caroline Creed, our ever-helpful editor at William Heinemann Medical Books.

Chapter 1

The Acute Dental Problem

PULPITIS

This condition produces sharp, poorly localised pain which can be of considerable severity. The site may be confused between the upper and lower jaws but is always on the same side. Pain is initially momentary and may be spontaneous or precipitated by hot, cold or sweet food. It becomes progressively more prolonged and may be related by the patient to recent treatment, injury (such as a cracked cusp), or occur in a tooth with a deep restoration.

Pulp vitality can be tested by applying a cold stimulus, e.g. a pledget of cotton-wool soaked in ethyl chloride, to the crown of a tooth, or an electrical pulp tester may be used on the dried tooth. In each instance the results should be compared with a healthy opposite tooth. Occasionally a tooth with pulpitis will be sensitive to percussion. Beware multirooted teeth in which one section of the pulp is moribund but the other area responds normally.

If pulpitis is early and recovery is thought possible, then the exposed dentine needs to be covered by a sedative dressing (eugenol-containing compounds are often successful), and this must obtund the exposed dentine. Where the exposure of an apparently healthy and bleeding pulp has occurred in the absence of gross contamination, pulpotomy in a young tooth, or pulp capping in the adult using calcium hydroxide dressings may enable continued pulp vitality. The pain of acute pulpitis may be temporarily controlled by the application of a dressing containing a steroid and an antibiotic.

Treatment requires the pulp to be anaesthetised (general anaesthesia may be required) and the removal of the pulp or the tooth itself. Pulpectomy should be followed by root canal obliteration as soon as the canal is clean and dry (at the first visit if the pulp is vital). Once canal preparation is complete, a variety of durable sealants may be used, care should be taken that these do not pass beyond the apex of the tooth. To form the bulk of the root filling, substances such as gutta percha may be inserted to occupy the central canal volume and ensure that the sealant is put under gentle pressure.

PERIODONTITIS

This is often described as a dull and continuous ache, and may become momentarily severe where pressure is applied to the involved tooth. Initially pressure on the tooth may allow transient relief of pain but eventually the patient will avoid any movement of the tooth or occlusal pressure whatsoever and will usually chew on the opposite teeth. The pain is characteristically well localised to one tooth which is highly sensitive to percussion. Physical exercise may well worsen the pain and produce an additional feature of continuous throbbing. Whenever numerous upper posterior teeth are sensitive to percussion, exclude maxillary sinusitis.

If the periodontitis is of traumatic origin it can often be relieved initially by removing the tooth from any occlusal pressure and correcting any 'over-eruption' which may have occurred. If the tooth itself is sensitive to the high speed drill then the opposing tooth may be adjusted to lightly relieve the occlusion in all possible directions of contact. Local anaesthesia in these instances is characteristically difficult to achieve. If it is thought that an element of infection is likely, such as periodontitis following pulp death, then pain control will be assisted by an appropriate antibiotic prescription providing that treatment of the underlying infective cause is subsequently put in hand. Occasionally extraction of the tooth under a general anaesthetic may be required where symptoms prove difficult to control.

ALVEOLAR OSTEITIS

This often presents as severe, persistent, dull throbbing pain which is usually localised to the site of a recent infection or extraction but may, however, initially prove difficult to pinpoint and can radiate from the original site, e.g. to the ear from a lower third molar socket. It may well be that the alveolar osteitis is limited just to a recent extraction socket (dry socket). In this case, pain may be of a crescendo nature, aching in type, generally severe, and often occurring within 48 hours of an extraction (commonly of a lower molar). The socket is characteristically empty with denuded bony walls, and it should be ensured that no root fragments remain before commencing treatment. A variety of remedies (essentially topical and obtundant) have been advocated, including BIPP pack, zinc oxide and eugenol, Alvogyl, after first irrigating and cleansing the socket.

Prophylactically, follow basic principles of good oral hygiene, atraumatic extractions and proper haemostasis. Some systemic antibiotics, e.g. metronidazole have been shown to be effective. Signs that the osteitis is progressing include pyrexia in a fatigued patient where there is evidence of a previous infection. Additional features which should be of concern include numbness in the lower lip, features similar to sinusitis in the upper jaw and a progressively worsening pain affecting a more diffuse area.

Postoperative Pain

Management depends on the patient's perception in terms of severity, duration, mood and expectations, and the visible evidence of surgical treatment. The best course to adopt is to *prevent* pain before it becomes troublesome by early prescription and administration of adequate analgesics according to the scale of surgery. In the case of an out-patient treated under local anaesthesia this involves giving them oral analgesics or advising them to take such drugs before the anaesthetic effect is lost. The in-patient may be treated with injectable analgesics (narcotics if necessary) in order to prevent the experience of worse pain immediately postoperatively. Such initial measures *must* be followed by regular analgesic top-ups as required, and not given on a rigid (e.g. 6-hourly) regimen. For in-patients with severe pain, postoperative analgesic infusions using a small pump is a reliable method of administering effective, continuous analgesia, while avoiding peak and trough effects. In addition total dosage is considerably reduced. The fear of pain increases analgesic needs and impairs effectiveness. Prevention by early adequate analgesia is preferable.

PARAORAL 'FASCIAL SPACE' INFECTIONS

Following events such as pulpitis, periodontitis, pericoronitis and trauma, infection may progress into any nearby fascial plane or potential tissue space as shown in Figure 1.1(*a*) and (*b*). While each of these has characteristic features which will be described, *all* of them have a *general pattern* of presentation and progress, and it is these general features which will be discussed first.

The healthy adult without any effective antibiotic treatment will report progressively severe, dull, relentless pain often throbbing in nature and frequently associated with increasing stiffness in the jaw

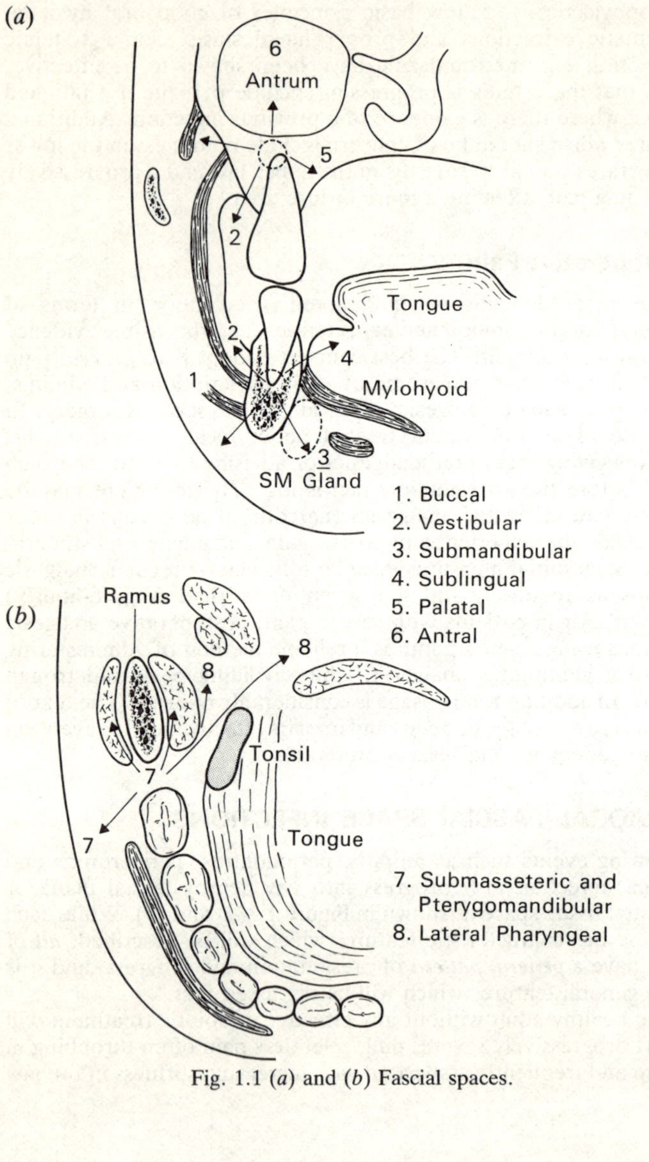

Fig. 1.1 (*a*) and (*b*) Fascial spaces.

and usually associated with swelling of the affected area. The patient may become quickly feverish and the temperature may show high transient peaks. Enlargement of the swelling may well be associated with reduction in local pain as pus breaks through some anatomical barrier.

Learn to assess the patient's *general condition* and progress from such indicators as severe or worsening pain, spiking temperature chart (probably indicating pus collection) and whether the patient appears 'clinically' ill with pallor, tiredness, anorexia, malaise and flushing. This involves an overall assessment from the end of the bed before considering minutiae, such as the causal tooth.

The principles of management are similar whatever fascial space is infected. In essence these comprise admission, bed rest, analgesics, hydration and parenteral antibiotics (of a suitable agent in bacteriocidal doses). Consider early drainage if there is pus collection. To drain an abscess externally a skin incision is made at a dependent point over the swelling and preferably in a skin crease. Plan to avoid underlying vital structures, such as main vessels and nerves. Thereafter blunt dissection by introducing sinus forceps, opening and withdrawing them may proceed down towards the suspected origin of the infection until pus is located, or the deepest of the expected structures is encountered, e.g. mandible. As soon as pus is found, good samples should be obtained (swab plus a syringe specimen preferably). The cavity is explored to rupture any further locules of pus, and a suitable drain (e.g. corrugated plastic) is introduced into the abscess cavity and sutured into position. An absorbant dressing pad is applied and fixed over the wound and should be changed every 24 hours, or as soon as it is outwardly stained. When the wound stops discharging the drain may be shortened, 2.5 cm at a time until ineffective, when it is removed.

Since abscess drainage often requires general anaesthesia you will need to assess the patient's fitness both for general anaesthesia and for endotracheal intubation if the abscess is close to the oropharynx or if trismus has been present for more than 7 days. If a general anaesthetic is planned then clearly the opportunity to remove the cause of the infection may well present itself. The choice is between early operation for drainage against a few hours' delay to rehydrate a sick patient and commence high dose antibiotics to control the systemic effects of infection. The choice of antibiotic regimen (which may be multiple) is urgent and important, requires experience and is worth discussing with your senior clinician should there be any doubts about drug selection. The patient will require regular checks on clinical progress at a frequency determined initially by their clinical condition, and subsequently by the rate of improvement. Discharge from the ward should be considered when their clinical condition is clearly improving reliably, they have been apyrexic for 48 hours, oral fluids are being taken comfortably, and appetite has returned together with subsiding pain levels.

Considering individual sites of infection (see Fig. 1.1(*a*) and (*b*) p. 4), the specific clinical presentation of space infections is outlined as follows.

Buccal

There is tender swelling above and lateral to body of the mandible often near the root of a causal tooth. If the infection is *not* deep to platysma the skin will often redden quickly and any pus which forms will burst through the surface more easily and drain spontaneously, an event which should be forestalled by incision and drainage as soon as signs of pus collection are present.

Vestibular

The swelling covered only by mucosa will present earlier signs of fluctuance, but may not always present opposite the causal tooth. Incision across the sulcus and drainage by blunt dissection are usually straightforward and should be considered under local anaesthesia in the first instance, even though the presence of infection might well preclude removal of a causal tooth. Beware of the mental nerve.

Submandibular

There is diffuse tender swelling associated with dysphagia deep to the platysma and body of the mandible in the upper neck. Bimanually palpable on the cutaneous side of the mylohyoid muscle, late to 'point'. It may well spread beneath the platysma inferiorly to the lower neck or posteriorly towards the pharynx. Usually this tissue space infection is limited from further medial spread to the submental space by the digastric muscle. Wide mouth opening is painful and elevation of the tongue is not a feature. Drainage should be via a neck crease incision below the surface markings of the cervical branch of the facial nerve, carefully avoiding the facial vessels during exploration.

Sublingual

A lower tooth with its apex above the mylohyoid muscle attachment and from which pus 'points' lingually may well produce cellulitis and abscess formation in this area. It is characterised by painful swelling under one side of the tongue which becomes progressively raised. This is associated with dysphagia and should the infection spread into the submandibular space and across the midline, the features of incipient Ludwig's angina will be witnessed with considerable systemic 'toxaemia' and concomitant hazard to the airway. When intraoral incision for drainage of the sublingual space is planned the operator must keep in mind the course of the lingual nerve, Wharton's duct and posteriorly the facial vessels.

Lateral Pharyngeal

Infection between the tonsil and the medial pterygoid muscle will produce considerable pain, dysphagia, systemic disturbances and intense trismus. A variable degree of swelling in the lateral pharynx may be evident, also externally at the angle of the mandible. Careful assessment is essential with regard to the hazard of pus spillage into the pharynx during induction of general anaesthesia and intubation of the trachea in the presence of trismus. If this seems at all likely, precautions must be taken to avoid tracheal soiling. For drainage, care in choosing the incision site is important as is proper exploration of all recesses which extend superiorly to the infratemporal region, and adequate anchorage of any drain or pack put into the infected space is likewise essential.

Submasseteric and Pterygomandibular

Several features of infection in these two 'spaces' are similar, notably intense trismus, minimal external swelling, considerable pain and systemic effects. The affected overlying muscle is tender and in spasm and there may be high fever. Clinical suspicion is particularly important and drainage of such pus collection under general anaesthesia can be approached intraorally via an incision along the ascending ramus of the mandible and suitable exploration lateral or medial to the rami.

Palatal

Subperiosteal abscesses may well stem from palatally placed roots of lateral incisors, premolars or molars and be of apical or periodontal origin. Drainage is usually easy to establish and can be achieved under local anaesthesia, bearing in mind the blood vessels from the palatine and nasopalatine foramina. A drain is rarely required, if necessary a window of palatal mucoperiosteum may be excised to allow continuing drainage.

PERICORONITIS

This can affect the soft tissues of any incompletely erupted tooth, the vast majority of cases affecting the lower third molars. A mixture of gingival trauma, poor oral hygiene, oral infection elsewhere (acute ulcerative gingivitis), poor gingival configuration, certain systemic conditions (diabetes, pregnancy, upper respiratory infections) and sometimes seasonal influences (autumnal) all combine to produce inflammation of the pericoronal tissue. This may become established and spread. Depending on its site, adjacent structures affected by spreading infection will produce local effects initially; in the case of a lower third molar these include soreness, cheek trapping, bad taste, trismus and difficulty in chewing. The condition is often mild, recurrent and may resolve spontaneously, until a severe or persistent episode leads to cellulitis and infection of nearby 'tissue spaces' as outlined previously in this chapter.

Pericoronitis alone may often be controlled by removing any traumatising opposing cusps (including a functionless upper third molar), giving oral hygiene instruction, hot saline mouthwashes and analgesics. More specific measures include the careful application of caustics to the pericoronal tissues to hasten shrinkage, obtund and provide local antisepsis. Extreme care is advised in the use of agents, such as silver nitrate or trichloracetic acid and they must be chemically neutralised with suitable agents, e.g. glycerol, and copious water irrigation provided. If the patient shows evidence of systemic effects or spreading infection (pyrexia, sleep loss, severe trismus, lymphadenitis) then it would be wise to prescribe systemic antibiotics, to review after 24 hours and when settling, to discuss prevention of recurrent attacks, often by removal of the causal tooth.

Chapter 2

Maxillofacial Injuries

The general principles of managing patients admitted with acute injuries, including facial trauma, may be considered under four headings.

IMMEDIATE MANAGEMENT

Establish and Maintain a Clear Airway

(1) Clear debris from the mouth (dentures, broken teeth etc.), suck out the blood and saliva and insert a nasal or oral airway if necessary; a tracheostomy is only rarely required.
(2) Turn the patient on his side (other injuries permitting).
(3) Keep suction apparatus to hand, with an assistant available to use it, in case vomiting occurs.
(4) An anaesthetist may be required to insert an endotracheal tube.

Control of Haemorrhage

Severe bleeding is only rarely a problem in maxillofacial injuries. The use of external pressure, packing or suturing is often sufficient to gain immediate control. Bleeding into the chest or abdomen poses a much greater threat to the patient and must be recognised early.

Treatment of Shock (see also Chapter 19)

For practical purposes, shock is defined as hypoperfusion of vital organs. If systolic blood pressure below 100 mmHg and a pulse rate above 100 beats/min occurs insert an intravenous cannula and commence fluid replacement.

Initial Care of Injuries

Hard tissue injuries may require temporary immobilisation (splints or bandaging) and sterile dressings if compound. Soft tissue injuries may need temporary taping (Steristrips) or loose suturing.

This sequence is carried out in the first few minutes, usually in the casualty department. The patient is kept nil by mouth until definitive treatment has been planned.

GENERAL AND SPECIFIC EXAMINATION

The patient is now stabilised, vital signs are monitored and full clerking of the patient commenced.

Initial cardiovascular records should include blood pressure and pulse rate monitoring at frequent intervals until the patient is clinically stable. Electrocardiogram (ECG) monitoring is often required. Central venous pressure recording may be particularly useful if large fluid replacement is commenced. Peripheral perfusion of the limbs should be watched if limb injury is present.

Now that the upper airway has been established, the chest should be examined clinically, careful auscultation and percussion being carried out. A chest radiograph is often required to exclude injury to the lungs and ribs.

Attention should be given to the neurological status of the patient, since many maxillofacial injuries have an associated cranial or spinal injury. Three baseline observations must be recorded at the earliest opportunity.

(1) The level of consciousness may be recorded using the Glasgow Coma Scale (see Appendix F., p. 203).

(2) Reaction and size of the pupils.

(3) Other abnormal neurological signs.

Particular care is directed towards any deterioration of the neurological state. Investigations, such as CT scanning, may be appropriate and early specialist opinion sought should doubt exist as to further management.

If the patient is conscious on admission, the history of the accident and his own medical history should be obtained. Should the patient be unconscious, ambulance men or other witnesses should be questioned. Telephone the patient's doctor if clarification of the patient's medical history is required.

INVESTIGATIONS

The investigations ordered depend on the results of the history and examination. In maxillofacial injuries appropriate investigations may include radiographs of the skull and facial skeleton, haematological investigations, e.g. tests including haemoglobin level, packed cell volume, sickle cell index (Sickledex), crossmatching and biochemical tests, such as the monitoring of electrolyte balance.

At this point, appropriate specialist opinions are sought and definitive treatment is planned.

DEFINITIVE TREATMENT

When sufficient information has been gathered by the relevant medical attendants, further treatment is planned, giving due weight to the medical priority of each injury. The timing of surgery is dependent upon the patient's clinical condition.

It is at this point that the patient's relatives should be fully informed of the patient's injuries and proposed treatment.

MANAGEMENT OF FACIAL LACERATIONS

(1) *Wound cleansing*—Locate and remove foreign bodies, such as root fragments or glass. Dirt tattoo removal may have to be carried out.
(2) *Conservation of soft tissue*—Only obviously necrotic tissue should be removed. Replace tissue to its original anatomical position. Z-plasties are seldom indicated in a primary repair, but wound margins may require revision or undermining before approximation. Extensive soft tissue loss requires specialised expertise.
(3) *Suture selection*—Select appropriate suture material, e.g. 5/0 monofilament for skin, 3/0 plain catgut for subcuticular use and 3/0 silk for mucosal repair.
(4) *Timing of suture removal*—Alternate facial sutures may be removed on the 4th day, the remainder being removed one day later. Steristrips may help support the wound if wound dehiscence is feared. Intraoral sutures are usually removed after a week.
(5) *Wound closure*—Soft tissue injuries should generally be sutured within 24 hours. Fracture reduction and fixation should precede repair of facial lacerations.
(6) *Check antitetanus prophylaxis.*

EPISTAXIS

This may be spontaneous or in response to trauma. If epistaxis proves difficult to stop, crossmatch the patient's blood and insert a drip. This often occurs in elderly, atherosclerotic and hypertensive patients. It may unveil a bleeding disorder and thus a clotting screen may be indicated. The bleeding often occurs from Little's area on the antero-inferior part of the nasal septum.

Management

(1) Estimate blood loss and take baseline blood pressure and pulse measurements.
(2) Pinch nose between thumb and forefinger for 5 minutes.
(3) If bleeding persists suck out blood from nose and inspect cavity using a Thudicums nasal speculum and a bright light. An obvious bleeding point requires cautery.

If bleeding is still a problem insert a nasal pack—suck blood from the nose, spray with lignocaine and wait 2 minutes. Cut the index finger off a standard surgical glove (approximate size 6) and pack with 2.5 cm ribbon gauze. Lubricate with a smear of KY jelly and gently insert into the nose using non-toothed forceps. Insert a safety pin through the exposed end to prevent the pack passing posteriorly. Remove after 24 hours.

INJURED AND LUXATED TEETH

Injuries to teeth occur in isolation or in association with bone and soft tissue injury. Clinical examination and X-rays assist in injury classification. The appropriate treatment, as in Table 2.1, can then be arranged.

Injuries to the Deciduous Teeth

These injuries include:

Avulsions—generally not treated.
Subluxation—splinting is difficult, hence 'watch and see' policy.
Intrusion—most common. If less than 75% of crown is intruded, leave to erupt.

Possible sequels to trauma include pulp death or opacity due to calcification, pink spot because of internal resorption, ankylosis or relative submergence.

Effects on the underlying permanent dentition include discoloration of enamel, enamel hypoplasia, crown dilaceration, formation of odontome and root duplication.

Table 2.1
Injuries to the Permanent Teeth

Classification	*Injury to tooth*	*Treatment notes*
Class I	Enamel chipping only	Smooth enamel ? composite restoration
Class II	Coronal fracture involving enamel and dentine only	Cover exposed dentine, e.g. $Ca(OH)_2$ ± temporary crown
Class III	Coronal fracture exposing pulp	If root has an open apex, carry out a pulpotomy and cover with $Ca(OH)_2$ and zinc oxide/eugenol dressing. If apex closed, extirpate pulp and root fill.
Class IV	Root fracture ± coronal fracture	Depends on the position of the fracture. Apical third fracture may require root extirpation ± splinting. Other fractures generally indicate extraction.
Class V	Displaced tooth	If sufficient periodontal support, reinsert at the earliest opportunity and consider splinting, e.g. wiring or acid-etch to adjacent teeth.

SPLINTING OF TEETH

Teeth may be effectively splinted by either of two simple techniques.

'Vacuum Soft Acrylic Splint'

Take an alginate impression of the teeth requiring splinting (often simply achieved by a whole arch impression) and have a 'vacuum soft acrylic splint' made. This can be cemented with zinc oxide and eugenol.

Wiring

A single wire (approximately 0.3–0.4 mm stainless steel) is passed around an adjacent tooth (or teeth) either side of the tooth (teeth) to be splinted. This is tightened. Interdental wiring involves wires placed as loops on either side of the tooth to be splinted, the loop is then tightened.

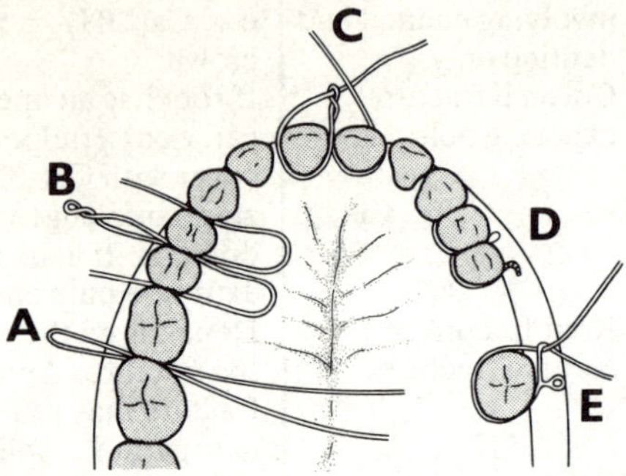

Fig. 2.1 (*a*) A,B,C stages in routine eyelet wiring. E, method using soldered eyelet on lone-standing teeth. To stabilise a mobile tooth place wires around tooth on either side and tighten.

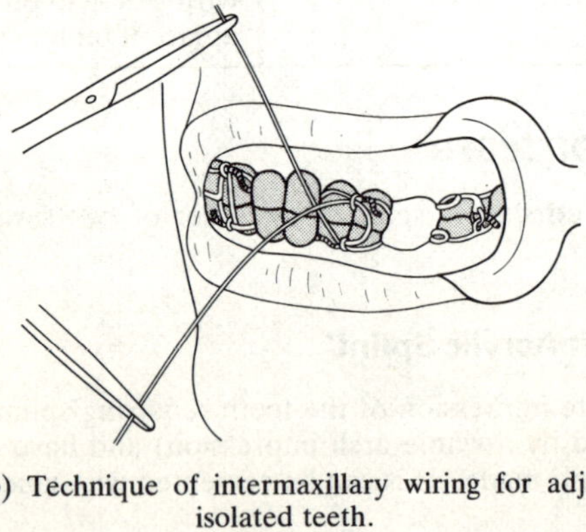

Fig. 2.1 (*b*) Technique of intermaxillary wiring for adjacent and isolated teeth.

FRACTURES OF FACIAL BONES

It is often the most junior member of the hospital team who is first asked to see the 'casualty patient'. He will be required to make the immediate assessment and to commence the management of the patient. The general principles of fracture management for facial fractures involve reduction, immobilisation and fixation.

Aetiology of Facial Injuries

Facial injuries result mainly from fights, sporting injuries, falls and road traffic accidents (RTAs). Alcoholic intake is a common finding in patients in these categories. The aetiology of the injury may have clinical significance, e.g. RTAs often involve litigation, fights may involve the police.

Immediate Care

The immediate management has been outlined at the beginning of this chapter.

History

A concise history of the accident (from the patient or his attendants) should be obtained together with details of his medical history. The patient's general medical history may have bearing on his management, e.g. history of diabetes mellitus, chronic alcoholism or drug abuse.

Clinical Examination

This should consist of a general physical examination of all the major systems, with the patient's clothes removed. Male housemen examining female patients require a chaperone.

In addition, a specific examination of the injured site(s) is mandatory. Accurate records of the history and examination at the time the patient is first seen are extremely important in preparing reports required for any subsequent litigation.

Initial Management

At this point sufficient information should have been obtained to enable you to gauge:
(1) The severity of the injury.
(2) Whether other medical/surgical teams need to be involved.
(3) Whether the patient requires hospital admission.
(4) What investigations are required.
If any doubt exists on any of these points, ring your immediate superior and request advice.

If the patient is to be admitted and an operation is planned in the near future, the patient is kept starved. Pain relief may be required. An intravenous infusion might be appropriate at this point.

Investigations

The definitive diagnosis of facial fractures largely depends on good radiographs. If the patient is unconscious, restless or drunk, definitive radiographs may be best obtained at a later time. Useful X-rays for facial fractures include an OPG, PA of the skull, O–M views, lateral skull views together with intraoral films to show fractures of teeth or the alveolus.

Other investigations may be appropriate and are similar to an admission for a routine operation (see Chapter 5).

Timing of Surgery

The reduction of facial fractures is rarely required immediately. Factors which should be taken into consideration when planning definitive surgery include:
(1) History of loss of consciousness—Monitor neurological state. Twenty–four hours is usually allowed to elapse before surgery is contemplated.
(2) Availability of theatre time, anaesthetist and other surgeons.
(3) Sufficient time to plan the surgery and arrange the technician to make arch bars, splints, etc.
(4) Stomach emptying should be complete—Usually 6 hours since ingestion of food.
Make sure that the patient and his relatives understand the diagnosis and the planned surgery; 5 minutes of friendly explanation may remove hours of anxiety for the family.

Planning the Treatment of the Fractures

While the responsibility for final planning of the surgery may not be in your hands, an intelligent assessment at an early stage is required. Factors which are taken into the overall equation include:
(1) Age and general health of the patient.
(2) Position, number and severity of the fracture(s).
(3) Dental status, i.e. number of teeth present and the periodontal condition.
Useful guideline: 'Pathology' present in the fracture line, e.g. fractured teeth, retained roots, cysts or foreign bodies must be removed, or delayed union, non-union or persistent infection are risked.

Upper and lower impressions may be required to determine the correct occlusion. If the fracture(s) has/have produced a step in the occlusion, either the models will have to be split or impressions can be taken with half trays, and the impressions joined by the technician.

Notes on Types of Fixation

(1) *Eyelet wiring with intermaxillary fixation (IMF)*—Usually appropriate for simple fracture(s) with an intact dentition.
(2) *Arch bars with intermaxillary fixation*—The arch bars may be custom-made for the individual patient on the patient's dental model, or preformed. They are used where extra rigidity is required, e.g. where teeth are missing, teeth are periodontally involved, or bilateral fractures are present.
(3) *Silver cap splints with intermaxillary fixation*—Made by the technician, may be sectioned or of full arch coverage. They are cemented on preoperatively and may be used in conjunction with extraoral fixation.
(4) *Gunning splints*—May be used in edentulous patients. Impressions can be obtained using the patient's full dentures, if they are intact.
(5) *Transosseous wiring*—May be used in addition to the methods described above.
(6) *Bone plating*—This has several advantages including that of immediate rigidity. Bone plating may be appropriate in the management of epileptics or other medically compromised patients, where the jaws do not necessarily have to be wired together.

Immediate Postoperative Care

(1) For all patients—Monitoring of the cardiovascular and respiratory systems (see Chapter 4).
(2) For patients in intermaxillary fixation—Check wire cutters accompany the patient. Instruct the nurses on how to cut the wires in an emergency. Suction apparatus should be available.
(3) Where surgery has been performed around the orbits the great danger is the rare problem of a retrobulbar haemorrhage. Warning signs are increasing pain in the eye, proptosis, decreasing visual acuity and loss of pupillary reflexes.
(4) Prescribe fluids (intravenous, nasogastric routes, etc.). Write up immediate analgesia and antiemetics (see Chapter 1). Consider whether antibiotics are required.

Postoperative Mouth Care

(1) Aim—A clean, healthy mouth to promote early healing.
(2) Regular toothbrushing—Soft brush.
(3) Mouth rinsing—Four to five rinses daily with chlorhexidine solution or warm salty water.
(4) Freedom from discomfort—Turn in wires, provide patient with soft wax, etc.

Follow-up Appointments

(1) Arrange regular appointments—Check occlusion, fixation and removal of sutures, etc.
(2) Estimate approximate time in fixation—This will depend on many factors.
(3) Final appointment—Allow sufficient time for the removal of fixation, cleaning of the teeth and final radiograph(s).

Medico-legal Considerations

(1) Keep accurate records—Initial history and examination, operation notes and details of follow-up.
(2) Obtain photographs.
From the above, solicitors and police reports can be drafted, often by someone else many months later (see Chapter 20).

Chapter 3

The Out-patient Clinic

THE APPROACH

Remember above all that your patient is a person in need of help or advice. Therefore always exercise a humane approach with additional tolerance if the patient has a problem, e.g. dysarthria. Initially, quickly assess the patient's hearing, intelligence and comprehension, and remember that they may be particularly anxious or may have prepared comments they wish to make.

Guide the history positively with carefully chosen questions to elicit significant points and responses. Adopt a positive approach and if you are uncertain about any points raised, ask another clinician early on.

RELATIONSHIPS

Clinical Colleagues

Ask for advice when puzzled by clinical or organisational matters, but choose your moment. Always ask for help at an early stage if you are having difficulty coping with the volume of work, or with a particular problem that you are unable to sort out.

Staff

Learn to get help and cooperation from the staff. Exercise the art of diplomatic delegation enabling others to become involved in the smooth running of the clinic so that they feel an essential part of the team. Watch and listen and, as far as possible, do not cause upheaval of the existing framework.

Organisation/Clinical Efficiency

(1) Get there early.
(2) Keep to appointment times, as far as is feasible, and apologise briefly if you have kept a patient waiting.

(3) Check the patient's notes before the clinic, read them through and familiarise yourself with them.
(4) Other matters should be dealt with before you appear at the clinic, e.g. telephone calls and ward checks. Make sure that casualty is clear and arrange for outstanding tasks to wait.
(6) Determine from the referral letters which patients need radiographs before they are seen, prepare their request cards, and ask your nurses to check whether women are likely to be pregnant.
(7) Anticipate being delayed by prolonged surgical cases. Attempt to see the patients with minor problems at a convenient moment, e.g. while waiting for the local anaesthetic to take effect.
(8) In the clinic, ask a nurse to complete the rubric on investigation or prescription forms. You may be fortunate in having an experienced nurse who can take blood samples for you, if that is the system in your hospital.
(9) Plan your own work to finish on time and to avoid obvious misjudgements, e.g. treating a patient requiring intravenous diazepam at the end of a busy clinic when they will require 1 hour to recover, or patients requiring intramuscular injections 30 minutes before a surgical appointment. Equally bear in mind important times such as when the pharmacy and X-ray department close. Likewise, anticipate the need for ambulance transport well in advance.
(10) At the end of the clinic leave instructions regarding patients who have not attended. They may need either contacting by telephone or sending a further appointment, or a letter to their general practitioner. Write notes regarding what was said to the patient, whether they were put on a waiting list, and discuss a course of action with your senior clinician at the earliest opportunity if this is your unit's policy.

Correspondence

If you are expected to do your own letters include the following:
(1) The clinic date.
(2) The name of the consultant under whom the patient was seen.
(3) Presenting history, diagnosis and treatment plan.
(4) What was said to the patient.
(5) Consider whether a copy need be sent to the patient's general medical practitioner or other involved hospital units. If a patient has already been seen about this or a closely related condition,

communication is important to avoid duplication of effort and to ensure that other clinicians are aware that you are seeing the patient.
These considerations are especially important if you are prescribing, if there is significant disease process, if general anaesthesia is planned, or if the past medical history is not clear.

PREOPERATIVE PROCEDURE IN THE OUT-PATIENT DEPARTMENT

(1) Check the diagnosis, past medical history and investigations.
(2) Anticipate the needs of the surgical team.
(3) Assess the suitability of the patient for anaesthesia and any special requirements needed.
(4) Ensure that appropriate radiographs are present (which would enable you personally to carry out the operation).
(5) Urinanalysis is advisable, and a full blood count is important before general anaesthesia.
(6) Include an electrocardiograph where the history indicates cardiovascular disease or the patient is over 60 years of age, or when major surgery is planned. Have to hand chest X-rays (posteroanterior) when there is a history of chest disease or if a rib graft is planned.
(7) Obtain informed consent (see Chapter 20).

Choice of Anaesthesia

This may include:
Local anaesthesia
Local anaesthesia plus sedation (intravenous/inhalation)
General anaesthesia.

Factors to Consider in the Choice of Anaesthesia

(1) The patient's demeanour, self-control, anxiety level, intelligence, squeamishness, level of comprehension of events and whether their general medical health is poor.
(2) The likely skill of the operator and anticipated duration of the procedure.
(3) The likelihood of operative problems/complications, e.g. access or major bleeding.

(4) Anticipate the need for techniques with poor patient acceptability such as chiselling or diathermy.

(5) Social background, home support, home distance, home transport availability, availability of adult escort, children at home needing attention, etc.

(6) Consider contraindications to general anaesthesia, such as patients who show myocardial insufficiency, diabetics, or the elderly. Anticipate the need for strong postoperative analgesia or an observation period, or the need for other prescriptions, e.g. hypoglycaemic, antihypertensive, cardiotonic or diuretic.

The choice of anaesthesia is controlled by the operator's preference, patient suitability, and your unit's policy. This is a general guide to important considerations, some of which will be of overriding concern in given instances, but if in doubt ask your senior clinician.

THE MEDICALLY COMPROMISED PATIENT (see also Chapter 19)

Angina or Recent Myocardial Infarction

(1) Patients with angina or recent myocardial infarction are best treated under local anaesthetic (LA) since general anaesthetic (GA) carries an operative mortality which is initially high after myocardial infarction, but declines exponentially after the event, and becomes almost normal 2 years later.

(2) Postpone non-essential treatment unless symptoms have or are likely to enforce an acute exacerbation.

(3) Full medical information about the infarct, complications, drug intake and present vital signs should be obtained.

(4) Avoid catecholamine containing LA but ensure adequate depth of anaesthesia as nothing raises endogenous catecholamines more than pain in a frightened patient. Consider additional intravenous diazepam if patient is anxious and their blood pressure is normal.

(5) Commence with sublingual glyceryl trinitrate 500 mcg preoperatively. However, vasoconstrictors injected locally may reduce its absorption.

(6) Adopt a calm, confident manner with regular reassurance and progress reports to the patient. Regularly check their general condition, colour, etc.

(7) Be prepared to put the patient back into a suitable position if angina or a vasovagal attack should supervene during treatment; if

consciousness is lost during a faint (pallor, initially slow or weak pulse, then tachycardia) tip the patient head down, check the pulse, and quickly reach a diagnosis as medical expertise may be required.

(8) Be prepared to allow the patient to rest during the procedure, and remember that the appointment for suture removal may be equally stressful for the patient as the operation itself.

Patients Taking Steroids

All patients receiving systemic corticosteroids within the preceding 18 months generally require steroid supplements before the operation. Clinically it is usual to assume a deficient endogenous response and the aim therefore is to administer sufficient corticosteroid during what is presumed to be a stressful period. Additional steroids should therefore be in circulation at the time of stress and subsequently be continued for an adequate period. If complications arise (infection or severe pain) then more and prolonged steroid supplement must be given.

Plan your patient's appointment so that they arrive 30 minutes before the operation, enabling your nurse to have the drug available, and give the patient the steroid injection intramuscularly on arrival and record the time. Alternatively you may prefer to administer the steroid intravenously if an indwelling cannula is in use for sedation or antibiotics.

It is wise to retain the patient for at least 30 minutes postoperatively for pulse/blood pressure recording and give clear instructions to the nurse on how to obtain help.

Also consider whether to provide antibiotic cover.

An adequate steroid regimen would be intramuscular or intravenous hydrocortisone 200 mg 30 minutes preoperatively. Reliable patients still on oral steroids can take instead an increased dose on the day of operation, decreased over 3 days:

Day of operation—twice (plus 100%) normal maintenance dose
Second day—1.5 times (plus 50%) normal maintenance dose
Third day—1.25 times (plus 25%) normal maintenance dose
Fourth day—resume normal dose

Patients requiring steroid supplements include those with rheumatoid arthritis, asthma, treated Cushing's disease, hypoadrenalism, serious dermatitis, connective tissue disorders, and those taking cytotoxic chemotherapy.

Patients at Risk from Oral Bacteraemia

In general, these patients need bacteriocidal antibiotic blood levels for procedures likely to cause a bacteraemia at the time of treatment to prevent infective sequelae elsewhere in the body, but more especially within the vascular system.

Formerly patients who had experienced rheumatic fever constituted the largest number but there are now several other categories in whom antibiotic cover is imperative; these are: patients with a history of cardiac/valvular/major arterial vessel disorder or surgery for these conditions; open heart surgery including coronary artery bypass; other arterial surgery (radial artery shunt for haemodialysis) and joint replacements. Such patients need a full history including details obtained from the cardiologist about drug intake, e.g. anticoagulants.

Define your treatment plan and bear in mind other treatments likely to produce a bacteraemia, which may be required in the foreseeable future. If feasible, it is better to condense treatments such as scaling, extractions, minor oral surgery and endodontics into one session to avoid the need to repeat courses of antibiotics and anticoagulant adjustment. However, it is essential to balance your enthusiasm with the patient's demeanour or frailty, and ask advice if you are uncertain.

Arrange an early appointment for antibiotic administration. Intramuscular antibiotics are ideal and should be commenced 30 minutes before treatment.

If necessary, and if bacteraemia may be prolonged, or sutures may cause a further bacteraemia, antibiotic cover can be continued until sutures are removed, one week later, or represcribed at that time. Remember to ask your patient postoperatively about any untoward systemic symptoms to exclude infective endocarditis.

Asthma or Poor Respiratory Efficiency

Any stress of an interview or minor surgical procedure under LA may worsen bronchospasm. Whereas most patients can tolerate some oral/pharyngeal pooling during minor oral surgery, the very dyspnoeic patient may not, and coughing may commence associated with cyanosis.

Remember most patients would prefer to sit erect and will not tolerate recumbency at all in view of increased dyspnoea. Remember

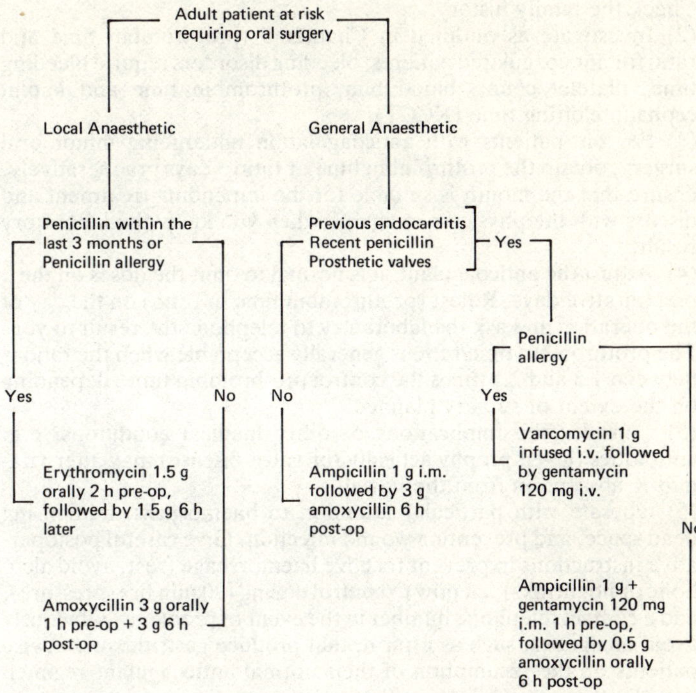

Fig. 3.1 Antibacterial endocarditis prophylaxis.

there may be drugs which will interact with those you are likely to prescribe and some chest diseases may require steroid supplements.

Anticoagulated Patient/Bleeding Diathesis

(1) The treatment plan must be well prearranged with advice from your senior clinician and other involved specialities including haematology and general medicine. Base your plan on a full history of past medical illness, e.g. stroke/valvular heart disease, paying particular attention to any bruising tendency, prolonged bleeding

from skin cuts, extraction sites or unusually frequent epistaxes etc. Check the family history.

(2) Investigate as outlined in Chapter 5 (prothrombin time and ratio for anticoagulated patients; bleeding disorders require bleeding time, platelet count, blood film, prothrombin time and kaolin cephalin clotting time (KCCT).

(3) For out-patients with anticoagulation undergoing minor oral surgery, obtain the prothrombin time or ratio 3 days preoperatively, ensure that the mouth is suitable for the impending treatment and discuss with the physician in charge when you know the laboratory result.

(4) Adjust the anticoagulant: it is normal to omit the doses on the 2 preoperative days. Retest (prothrombin time or ratio) on the day of the operation and ask the laboratory to telephone the result to you. The prothrombin time/ratio is generally acceptable when the ratio is between 1.5 and 2.3 times the control prothrombin time, depending on the extent of surgery planned.

(5) Consider the implications of other medical conditions, e.g. antibiotics (given prophylactically for valve disease) may alter vitamin K absorption from the bowel.

(6) Operate with particular attention to haemostasis, minimising dead space, and preventing wound infection. Give careful postoperative instructions to prevent reactive haemorrhage (rest, avoid alcoholic or hot drinks), on how to control oozing (20 min firm pressure), and a contact telephone number in the event of problems. Obviously avoid analgesics, such as aspirin, that produce gastritis, and advise patients on the resumption of their normal anticoagulant regimen (usually the normal dose on the day of operation).

(7) Liaise with the haematology department regarding the need for steroids, tranexamic acid or blood products, e.g. Factor VIII, plasma or fresh blood transfusions. Many of these products must be prepared freshly and given soon afterwards. Make allowances for the timing of treatment (usually earlier in the day) and the possible need for in-patient supervision. It is as well to keep the patient quiet, rested and with low anxiety level.

Patients with Poor Healing Response

These include patients undergoing radiation therapy, those on immunosuppressive drugs (including steroids) and those receiving haemodialysis.

(1) Anticipate complications from such treatments and provide prophylaxis.
(2) Treat all infections seriously and treat immediately.
(3) If possible avoid surgical extractions, or any bone-exposing techniques and minimise any infection-inducing process.
(4) Before treating, ask advice from the radiotherapist about the extent of any bony irradiation.
(5) If minor oral surgical procedure becomes inevitable, then the principles to be evoked are:
- (i) Minimise the amount of mucoperiosteum which must be stripped off (denudes blood supply).
- (ii) Operate efficiently and quickly.
- (iii) Suture carefully to avoid exposed bone or sharp, remaining spicules, as healing may be protracted and painful.
- (iv) Take additional precautions against secondary infection following treatment, by careful timing, good technique, meticulous wound toilet, topical preoperative antiseptics (0.2% chlorhexidine mouthwash), systemic antibiotics and postoperative observation to prevent haematoma.

(6) Consider the need to assess the area of ischaemic bone preoperatively by isotope scanning or radiographs and consider adjusting the doses of immunosuppressant drugs in conjunction with the controlling physician, e.g. cytotoxics reduced, steroids increased.

Patients with Hepatitis B or Acquired Immune Deficiency Syndrome (AIDS)

The situation regarding treatment of patients with antibody to the AIDS virus (HTLV III/LAV) is being constantly updated. Present recommendations are that patients who are *ill* with AIDS (or hepatitis B) should receive dental treatment in hospital. However, patients who are otherwise *well*, although presumed to be infectious, may be treated in general dental practice. Most carriers of blood borne viral diseases (including hepatitis B and AIDS) are not identified, and many receive routine dental treatment as a matter of course, as indeed they should, for the treatment of known carriers would not add materially to the hazards of practice. The transmissibility of HTLV III is low, there is felt to be little risk to health care workers, and no special provision of *non-clinical* areas is needed (e.g. waiting room, toilets).

Organising treatment for patients likely to transmit hepatitis B

(1) Be aware of the groups more likely to harbour hepatitis B infection—drug abusers, male homosexuals, leukaemics, haemophiliacs, patients on haemodialysis or those with Down's syndrome as well as Far Eastern patients. Until you *know* their infectivity status, take full protective precautions, expose the minimum number of staff to any potential risk. All staff should avoid contamination with blood or secretions.
(2) Try to handle the acute condition conservatively, perhaps using analgesics, antibiotics or a local dressing.
(3) Submit tests for infectivity status such as presence of HBs and HBe antigens and antibodies.
(4) As a general rule, all such cases, when potentially infective, should be treated at the end of a clinical session, using careful techniques, disposable equipment and protective clothing (double gloves, gown, cap, masks, goggles).
(5) Avoid the use of aerosol-producing sprays or hand-pieces. Surgical disposables should be incinerated in appropriate containers where possible; do not re-sheath needles. All affected items of equipment should be cleaned with glutaraldehyde, disposed of in clearly labelled containers and if re-usable, should be fully autoclaved or soaked in fresh 2% glutaraldehyde for 3 hours. Non-disposable aspirator components and work surfaces should be cleaned with 2% glutaraldehyde, and silicone based impressions may be left in 2% glutaraldehyde for 1 hour with good effect.
(6) All specimens from patients known to have transmissible viral infection should be appropriately bagged according to unit policy and labelled so that laboratory staff are forewarned of any hazard.
(7) Dental practitioners should be encouraged to treat patients for routine dental work after suitable testing and taking appropriate precautions. Obviously cover cuts and abrasions with a waterproof dressing before starting.
(8) In the event of you or the nursing staff breaching the skin with a contaminated instrument firstly wash out the wound immediately and vigorously with clear water. Take serum from that person, and from the patient (for assessment of their current infectivity status) and request guidance from the local microbiology laboratory regarding the need for immunoglobulin prophylaxis.

Diabetic Out-patients (see also Appendix C.)

These patients need to observe specified meal times and calorie requirements. More rigid adherence to these requirements is needed when oral hypoglycaemics are being taken, and are most important when insulin injections are used, whatever their duration of effect. Other systemic effects which should be borne in mind include accelerated cardiovascular diseases (hypertension, myocardial/cerebral infarction), impaired vision and renal function (drug clearance), and a greater tendency to develop infections (spontaneous and postoperative).

Time the consultation and treatment to allow for designated meal times and remember the blood sugar consequences of nausea and vomiting induced by your treatment and drugs, the effect of postoperative pain on the patient's appetite, especially if insulin or hypoglycaemic drugs have already been given earlier in the day. Bear in mind the need to retain adequate masticatory function postoperatively. Antibiotic prescription may justify reconsideration because of diabetes mellitus.

Beware out-patient treatment under general anaesthesia and admit the patient, preferably on the preoperative day. Forewarn the anaesthetist of the need for assessment and of your operative plan. Preanaesthetic starvation must be tempered with the need for all diabetics to have *some* insulin, and for this to be covered with adequate glucose (usually given intravenously). Your unit policy may well require you to involve the medical team, and it would be wise to inform them of the patient's admission. Place such patients first on the operating list to minimise potential delays in treatment. Take a blood sugar sample 1 hour preoperatively and to ask the laboratory to telephone the result to you before theatre. An intravenous infusion containing 5% dextrose will probably be required during operation, and soluble insulin in reduced dosage should be given, nowadays infusion pumps are a suitable form of delivery. A further blood sugar request and specimen should be sent towards the end of the operation to assess the patient's needs for the rest of the day (according to their likely activities and calorie intake). If possible, revert to a normal insulin regimen the day after operation. Mild *hyper*glycaemia during such treatment is usually acceptable. Remember that beta-blockade will mask many clinical signs of neuroglycopenia under general anaesthesia.

Chapter 4

The In-patient

ADMISSION PROCEDURE

General

Some general procedures are as follows:
(1) Check when the patients are normally expected on the ward and will be available to you with their records.
(2) If a patient requires urgent examination and/or investigation ask to see that patient first.
(3) Organise your day so that you are free to complete your administrative duties early. Allow time for investigations and for other clinicians to see the patient.
(4) Introduce yourself to the patient; adopt a friendly, progressive, business-like approach—Do not immediately sit on the end of their bed as if you have settled in for the afternoon!
(5) Plan ahead so that complex patients are seen first to allow for investigations during normal working hours.
(6) Avoid restricting nursing activity by asking for a chaperone too far in advance.
(7) Plan your rounds—Avoiding visiting and meal times.
(8) Ensure that you check the current presenting complaint, cardiorespiratory reserve and past medical history.

HISTORY

Firstly review the patient's existing records. Get quickly to the point of significant history avoiding irrelevant aspects. Stereotyped questioning may be unnecessary.

Briefly confirm the patient's presenting complaint, note any change relevant to the treatment planned. Record details and results of treatment relating to the presenting condition. The patient's past medical history should include previous serious illness, operations, present drug history and a note of allergies. Obtain information concerning the following, remembering to relate questions to the age and fitness of the patient and the severity of the proposed treatment:

(1) *Cardiovascular*—Consider exercise reserve, e.g. how many flights of stairs the patient can ascend without breathlessness, angina or chest pain. Ask about palpitations, swelling of the ankles, dizziness or chest pain relating to effort or anxiety. Can the patient lie flat without breathlessness?
(2) *Respiratory*—Does the patient have a cough? Is this continuous or spasmodic? Is it confined to the winter? Is the cough productive? Note quantity and colour of sputum—is it ever blood stained? Ask whether the patient is a smoker, and if so, how many cigarettes are smoked each day.
(3) *Gastrointestinal*—Ask the patient details concerning: appetite, weight constancy, abdominal symptoms and bowel habit, frequency and nature of bowel motions.
(4) *Genitourinary*—Obtain information concerning frequency or urgency of urination. Is nocturia, dysuria or haematuria present? Any unusual urinary odour? Note menstrual history in female patients and its present phase.
(5) *Neurological*—Is there any sensory loss or motor weakness at any site? Note balance, gait, memory, orientation—all normal? Carry out tests mentioned in Chapter 15 on the functioning and pathology of the cranial nerves.

Formal family and social history may not be needed, but this is one way of getting to know a patient, to help them relax, and for them to realise that you are interested in them as people.

EXAMINATION

Assess your patient in general. Is the patient clinically well or are there any obvious generalised clinical signs (cyanosis, pallor or jaundice)? Are they very anxious or unusually relaxed? If in doubt, ask advice or assistance from senior colleagues. They may wish to consult other specialities, e.g. general physicians. Look at the patient's hands as they will give clues regarding smoking, occupation, finger clubbing, skin and arthritic changes that you can observe while taking their pulse.

Examination of the Cardiovascular System

(1) Check radial pulse (rate, rhythm, volume, character).
(2) Check blood pressure (patient sitting).

(3) Is there pitting oedema of the ankles or sacrum?
(4) Recline the patient to 45 degrees and examine the chest.
(5) Note jugular venous pressure (just visible at the clavicle during full expiration).
(6) Palpate the apex beat (the most lateral, inferior point of the heart's impulse) normally in the mid clavicular line, fifth intercostal space. Are the apex beat and radial pulse synchronous?
(7) Learn to recognise normal first and second heart sounds.
(8) Are additional sounds audible in systole or diastole.
(9) Do additional sounds radiate into the precordium or neck vessels?
(10) When in doubt, seek expert advice—request assistance from the resident medical officer.

Examination of the Respiratory System

(1) Is the trachea central?
(2) Are neck movements and extension normal?
(3) Are chest expansion and resonance to percussion equal bilaterally?
(4) Compare the vocal resonance bilaterally (ask patient to say 'ninety nine').
(5) Learn to recognise normal inspiratory/expiratory (vesicular) breathing sounds. Note abnormal signs—crepitations (moist), rhonchi (whistling). Record their site, respiratory phase, and whether cleared by coughing.

Examination of the Abdomen

(1) Carry out inspection, palpation, percussion and auscultation.
(2) Note any scars, swellings or unusual markings, e.g. blood vessels.
(3) Is the abdomen soft and non-tender in all areas?
(4) Palpate the liver edge (normally in right hypocondrium during full inspiration).
(5) Is the spleen or either kidney palpable with bimanual examination?
(6) Are the hernial orifices intact when the patient coughs?

Examination of the Maxillofacial Region

(1) Check lymph nodes, thyroid gland, facial asymmetry.
(2) Note signs of injury, surgery and abnormal jaw movement.

(3) Ascertain that dental and oral condition is unchanged. Do existing radiographs represent the current condition? Perform additional investigations, such as tooth vitality and current radiographs.
(4) Check ears and eyes with otoscope and ophthalmoscope.

CONSENT

Obtain a current written consent (see Chapter 20). Be prepared to explain the wording of the consent form to the patient. Do not permit modification of the printed form. A non-technical explanation, including any likely complications, e.g. paraesthesia after removal of third molars, is helpful and mandatory.

CHECK LIST

Check that you have the current history of patient's presenting complaint, cardiorespiratory status and other relevant findings. Make sure that investigations have been completed (blood, radiographs), the consent form signed, the patient starved and the drugs charted.

ORGANISATION OF OPERATION

Regular Lists

(1) Name the consultant or operating surgeon, the date and start time.
(2) List cases in order.
(3) Record patient's name, ward, operation, and whether general or local anaesthesia is to be used.
(4) Ask the surgeon about his preferred order.
(5) Anxious, very young patients (? day stay) and diabetic patients are generally first. Grossly infected or trauma cases are usually last on list.
(6) Ensure the list is available for early distribution to all involved, wards, theatres, anaesthetic department, and that surgeons are informed.
(7) Inform theatre supervisor of any special requirements, such as plating set for fractures, amalgamator for apicectomies, or if operating list may be prolonged.

Urgent Lists

(1) Ascertain the preferred time of operation from your surgeon.
(2) Contact the theatre sister, inform her of the operation details, ask what other cases are booked and fix the theatre time.
(3) Consult the anaesthetist, who will visit and premedicate the patient.
(4) Advise the ward, who will prepare the patient.
(5) *If for any reason this plan changes, you must reinform everyone (theatre, surgeon, anaesthetist, ward—in that order)*, and ask the ward to inform the *patient* of any reason for delay.

THEATRE LORE

(1) Be early and ensure that the patient is sent down.
(2) Check notes and side and site of operation.
(3) Display radiographs and models.
(4) In theatre, sister is in charge.
(5) Use 'no touch' technique when scrubbed and stand out of the way, hands on your chest when not operating.
(6) If not assisting, be generally helpful (adjust the light, send for next case, convey messages clearly to the operating team).

SCRUBBING, GLOVING AND DRAPING

Aims

(1) To minimise the number of micro-organisms on the hands of the operating team (if glove puncture occurs).
(2) To cover the operating team and unoperated areas of the patient in sterile fabric to minimise risks of wound cross-infection.
(3) Once gowned, gloved and the patient draped, the operating team observe strict 'no touch' technique.
(4) Only sterile instruments are supplied as requested together with any surgical disposable.
(5) To allow a few minutes to discuss the planned surgical task.

Scrubbing Up

(1) Before starting, complete any last minute jobs, e.g. phone calls, make sure radiographs are displayed and that the usual operative requirements are available.

(2) Note the time and commence washing the hands and arms with soap two to three times, finishing on each occasion with rinsing under running water, draining from the elbows.
(3) Take a palm full of surgical scrubbing detergent, lather it on hands and arms, stopping at the elbow.
(4) Take a sterile brush without touching the brush holder using an elbow and the opposite hand, and methodically scrub all nails, then fingers and hands, and finally the arms, on the right and left side. Rinse the brush between different areas, discard it and finally rinse off the hands and arms again.
(5) Continue washing with surgical detergent, lathering fingers, hands and arms progressively and rinsing off until 3 minutes have passed, then rinse finally, allowing all free water to drain from the elbows into the scrub sink (not onto the floor).
(6) Turn off the tap with your elbows, move carefully to the gowning area—do not get behind people. Open your gown pack by grasping the inner fold without contaminating your hands, flatten it and take out the hand towel. When drying, do the hands first and finish near the elbows, being careful not to re-use a towel previously used near the elbow.
(7) Pick your gown, which will be folded inside out, grasp the shoulders by the inside, and shake it out without touching anything else. Hold the inside of each gown shoulder to assist your other arm through the sleeve. Your attendant will help you into the gown by handling only its inside surface and finish by tying the back.

Gloving

(1) When presented with your surgical gloves, grasp the inner packet without touching the outer cover, fold out the glove pack on the gowning surface.
(2) Take the talcum powder and liberally coat both hands (not gloved).
(3) Without touching the outer glove surface don the right glove by grasping its folded inside wrist surface with the left hand, then proceed as Fig. 4.1 (p. 36) shows.
(4) During the final turning back of the gloves to cover the gown cuffs, first fold over the gown cuffs and, with the opposite thumb pressing the folded cuff, use the opposite fingers to evert the glove over the gown cuff.

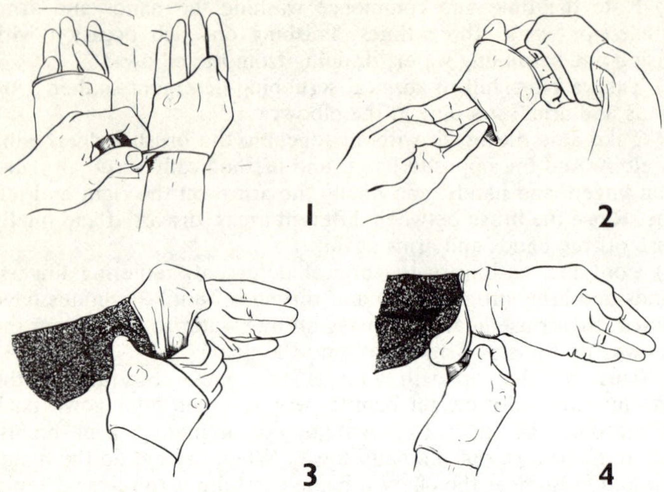

Fig. 4.1 Gloving procedure.

(5) Now fasten your waist tie by asking a scrubbed colleague to pass the tape round you. *From now on observe strict 'no touch' technique.*
(6) Stand, hands on chest to avoid contamination, in a quiet area of the theatre.

TOWELLING THE PATIENT FOR AN INTRAORAL PROCEDURE

Clearly, this towelling will be different for frontal, lateral facial or for neck procedures.
(1) Check the patient's position, e.g. neck extended for palatal procedure, or flexed for lower third molar.
(2) Ensure the anaesthetist is happy with the endotracheal tube, monitoring leads, intravenous infusion, and that any required diathermy pad or sand bags are *in situ*. Envisage the positions of the members of the operating team before positioning anaesthetic equipment.
(3) Sister will supply you with a container plus swab and sponge. Remember allergies occur with povidone-iodine antiseptic and avoid using spirit solutions near the eyes.

(4) Treat the area to be exposed thoroughly, plus a margin (say 5 cm) working centrifugally, then dry the treated area using the same method with a dry swab. Pass the antiseptic container to sister and give the discarded swabs to a nurse ('the runner').
(5) Towel the patient's head first. Use 2 medium squares superimposed, introduce these beneath the occiput to the neck while the anaesthetist flexes the neck (tube disconnected)—beware contaminating your gown or gloves. When the patient's head and tube have been restored to position, separate the upper towel each side and cross the towel below the nose leaving the lips exposed and clip the upper halves to each other where they cross at the patient's temple.
(6) Next pull up a long towel, bringing it up to the patient's neck covering the torso; this is clipped either side of the neck.
(7) Bring the table up to the operating height and if required help sister in preparing suction and drills for operation. Adopt an assistant's position.

ASSISTING

(1) Position yourself so that you can see well, and hold the retractors comfortably in the position where they are put by the operator.
(2) Avoid impairing the operator's movements and line of sight (to the wound, equipment and key personnel).
(3) Aspirate at a gravitationally dependent point in the wound, preferably on hard tissue (soft tissues block the aspirator tip).
(4) If asked to do something you are unsure of, say so.
(5) Ask if concerned by the patient's colour, diathermy function or some endangered vital structure.
(6) Be alert and anticipate the operator's next movement and be aware of difficulties encountered and act accordingly. Feed instruments and swabs back to sister if there is any problem with this.
(7) Cut sutures as directed and ensure that you can see well enough.

OPERATION RECORD

(1) Write in red ink on a specially designated sheet. Include the date, name of the surgeons, the assistants, the anaesthetist and the nurse in charge.

(2) As a general heading, enter an overall description of the operation, follow this by a succinct, detailed account of the procedure and findings.
(3) If you are unsure, ask.
(4) Sign the record and make a note of unusual recovery and ward instructions postoperatively, e.g. dressings, packs, additional drugs. Record blood loss and any operative complication.

WARD ROUNDS

These must be carried out regularly as often as required, each morning is generally a minimum. Ask the nursing staff if they are especially concerned about particular patients. Wear a badge with your name and position. It is your duty to explain things to the patient to allay their concern about their condition, treatment and their stay, and to reassure them.

Main Ward Round

(1) Ensure that the patient's notes, radiographs and investigation details are available before the round.
(2) Always ask the ward sister or her deputy for her permission to conduct a round, and preferably for her to accompany you.
(3) Brief the senior member of the round of any major, urgent or confidential problems before entering the ward.
(4) Lead the ward round to each patient and present a brief summary of the clinical case at the bedside, but avoid raising contentious issues within earshot of the patient. Mention the important investigation findings, including radiographs, where indicated.
(5) Conventionally, the member of the team conversing with the patient will stand close to the patient's bed on their right side, partly for examination purposes, with the senior nurse opposite.
(6) Record in the patient's notes what future management has been determined. If any doubts linger in your own mind regarding the next step and further management, clear them at the earliest opportunity with a more senior clinician.
(7) At the end of the round, check that sister or the nurse in charge is aware of the decisions that have been made.
(8) All laboratory reports should be seen and initialled daily.
(9) Watch the patient during the round lest comments have been misconstrued and if so return to the patient's bedside to clarify.

(10) When the patient is discharged from hospital inform both the general medical and dental practitioners of the treatment (in outline) in case their cooperation is needed.
(11) Learn the timetables of your consultant and senior registrar so that you can be prepared for ward rounds (or in case you need to contact them).

Business Round

(1) Establish a routine of rounds so that problems are pre-empted and the nurses know when management decisions will be taken and can plan their work. The early morning is ideal before the main day's work gets underway.
(2) For the first few days after major surgery (until ambulant) check observations of the patient's charted, pulse, blood pressure, temperature, etc.
(3) Check fluid balance, oral/i.v. fluid input versus fluid output (have they passed urine within 12 hours of operation?).
(4) Ensure that physiotherapy and drugs are being given.
(5) Record your findings in the notes.
(6) Before discharge, patients who have had a general anaesthetic need to be ambulant, looking after themselves, comfortable and trouble-free at the operation site.

PATIENT EXAMINATION

Examine the Patient's Chest

(1) Make enquiries concerning cough or sputum production.
(2) Possible cause of pyrexia after day 2.
(3) Each day look for poor unilateral chest expansion, percuss each lobar area (tap twice on the chest wall using the middle finger and the opposite hand), comparing the resonance of each side.
(4) Auscultate for breath sounds, rhonchi or crepitations and vocal fremitus (read about interpretation, e.g. an area with poor resonance, diminished breath sounds and coarse crepitations might well indicate lobar collapse).

Examine the Patient's Lower Limbs

(1) Inspect the calves of the patient, while they are lying on the bed, for symmetry, palpate for tenderness, especially at the inferior

aspect of the gastrocnemius muscle. Note any induration, prominent veins, poor perfusion or colour/temperature difference.

(2) Is Homan's sign present? (with the knee passively extended the ankle is firmly flexed to elicit calf tenderness).

(3) Deep venous thrombosis is often accompanied by a small temperature rise and usually follows long operations or in sick or immobile patients or in those with malignant disease.

Examine the Operation Wound

(1) Is there significant wound pain or bleeding, or problems related to posture?

(2) Remove the dressings, inspect and palpate the wound daily.

(3) Can drains be shortened or removed (according to duration and discharge)?

(4) Are vacuum drain bottles functioning?

(5) Do not wait for drains to become completely dry before removing them (1–3 days is usual).

(6) Instruct the nurses about further dressings (beware certain sites that the consultant may wish to keep covered for a finite period, e.g. skin grafts).

Dressings

(1) Remove dressings cautiously (? adherent), with antiseptic precautions if the wound is open.

(2) If the wound is open, redress using non-adhesive, absorbent material and if discharge is copious add a second absorbent layer.

(3) If repeated wound inspections may be needed, then use paraffin gauze for an initial layer to ease removal.

(4) Many surgeons prefer that dressings are removed after 24–48 hours and the wound left uncovered (unless clothing repeatedly irritates the area, e.g. iliac crest, or saliva or tracheal secretions contaminate the wound).

(5) Some surgeons prefer a sealant wound spray after removal of dressings.

Sutures

(1) Most intraoral sutures are silk and are removed at 5–10 days according to the clinical timetable or to wound progress.

(2) Catgut, Vicryl and dexon, being resorbable, are not generally removed.
(3) Monofilament nylon used for the skin is removed at 4–10 days (the finer the skin and the more visible the scar, the sooner they are removed).
(4) For all skin sutures, clean with antiseptic first, avoid stressing the wound traversely.
(5) With subcuticular sutures, pull one end, cut and remove by gently pulling the other end.

SKIN GRAFT-CARE OF DONOR SITE

If dressed conventionally with Sofratulle/paraffin gauze/absorbent pad, leave alone but tape it in place to prevent movement and for patient comfort. Check that it is not overtight and that the limb colour and peripheral perfusion is good. Soak off and inspect at 10 days. Usually there is a good dry graft bed, if this is so tape on a light non-adhesive dressing. If there is oozing from a thick graft donor site, reapply a non-adhesive dressing and observe at 2 day intervals. If there is excessive pain, pyrexia or local odour, soak off the dressing in a hot bath, but first ask your senior clinician. The donor site often looks tanned and may itch as a good graft heals; prescribe lanolin massage or lignocaine/calamine. Ask about the donor site at each visit in the early postoperative phase.

MORALE

How is the patient accepting the effects of the operation? Is the outcome as they expected? Look for signs of dismay or disappointment and talk to the patient about their future expectations and the future implications of the operation, such as when and how to plan their return to work.

POSTOPERATIVE PROBLEMS

Management of the Unconscious Patient in Recovery

(1) Close supervision by a trained, assigned person is essential until the patient is conscious (in full control of their own airway).
(2) Place the patient on their side (the tonsillar position) so that fluid drains dependently from the mouth, or is actively aspirated by

the assistant at intervals, until the patient is swallowing and able to protect their own airway.
(3) Ensure that suction, oxygen and assistance are available.

Bleeding

Bleeding when mild, will often respond to firm local pressure, e.g. from a swab rolled tightly and carefully pressed over the wound. After 15 minutes firm application, persistent, excessive or repeated bleeding will probably require attention. If it appears to be from the superficial layer, then try once more a further period of pressure using a warm pack before proceeding to the injection of a local anaesthetic plus vasoconstrictor, and opening of the wound to look for a bleeding point. Mattress sutures with generous tissue bites efficiently control superficial soft tissue oozing.

If only one site is troublesome, then, having excluded a bleeding vessel, a topical haemostatic agent, such as oxidised cellulose, may arrest further bleeding.

If a significant quantity of blood is being lost, and this appears to be from deep in the wound, then apply effective local pressure; ask your recovery nurse to continue this, discuss the problem with your senior clinician and arrange to replace significant blood loss. Where diligent local measures fail and other operative sites show a tendency to ooze, exclude a bleeding disorder (see Chapter 5). Consult your haematologist before requesting investigations.

Hypotension

Patients who do not sustain their usual blood pressure postoperatively need prompt investigation and attention. First assess the patient's conscious level, pulse rate, volume and regularity and whether they are warm and pink peripherally. Is the patient in a lot of pain and is the operation site satisfactory, or does it show signs of local bleeding or haematoma?

If the patient is dizzy when sitting, clearly he should be laid flat, and if necessary the bed tilted head down. Is the patient clinically dehydrated (dry tongue and mouth, loss of skin turgidity)? Consider the patient's fluid intake and loss over the last 24 hours, especially in very young and old patients who are more susceptible to dehydration.

The causes and treatment of postoperative hypotension are illustrated in Table 4.1.

Table 4.1
Causes and Treatment of Postoperative Hypotension

Problem	*Possible Causes*	*Investigation/Action*
Low cardiac output	Drug toxicity arrhythmia, infarct	ECG, medical opinion, appropriate measures
Poor peripheral arterial resistance	Drugs, posture, warm	Reverse cause
Venous pooling	Drugs, posture, congestive cardiac failure	Intravenous infusion, cardiotonics
Loss of circulating volume (bleeding, dehydrated)	Operation site, ? Bleeding elsewhere preop. starvation period, alcoholic unconscious after trauma	Intravenous infusion
Pain	Operation site, ? other injury	Adequate analgesia
Other predisposing causes	Previous hypotension (Malaysian/Mongoloid races)	Posture, keep in bed, consider elastic stockings

Patient Slow to Wake

(1) Check the vital signs (pulse rate + volume, blood pressure and peripheral perfusion, respiratory rate and depth). Ensure the patient is not just sleeping, having woken before. Check the pupils—diameter, reflexes and symmetry.
(2) Consider the length of operation, the anaesthetic agents already given, whether or not these are fully reversed.
(3) Was there any intraoperative hypotension, or respiratory obstruction?
(4) Has the patient had a myocardial infarct (ECG), a cerebrovascular accident (pupil reactions/limb movements) or is the patient excessively sedated postoperatively?
(5) If in doubt, ask the anaesthetist or his deputy and, in their absence, the medical registrar.

(6) Convey clearly to the ward sister the position in which you wish the patient to be under nursing attention, and frequency of observations required. If necessary request a special nurse.
(7) Postoperative nursing observations include conscious level, pulse, blood pressure, respiratory rate and wound attention.
(8) Special or major cases have individual requirements, e.g. major ablative operations, intermaxillary fixation, patients with intraoperative problems.

AIRWAY MANAGEMENT

Preventive

(1) Administer antiemetics, e.g. prochlorperazine (12.5 mg) or metoclopramide (10 mg i.v.) promptly.
(2) Avoid drugs likely to produce nausea, e.g. sweet elixir and opiates.
(3) Give pain relief and reassurance. However, beware of sedating anxious patients with poor airways.
(4) If the patient is nauseated, ask them to remain calm and to sit forwards with their elbows propped on a higher object, to take deep breaths and loosen their collar, and to call for help if they feel that they need it.
(5) Keep suction and oxygen by the bedside. If you anticipate major airway problems, as in nasal injuries which are packed and dressed, then it may be possible to arrange treatment of a lower facial injury without intermaxillary fixation, or to pass a nasopharyngeal tube. Ensure that this is patent by regular suction and check the air flow.
(6) Decongestant drops and inhalations may assist, especially where there is intermaxillary fixation.
(7) Practice endotracheal intubation with cooperative anaesthetists on operating lists.
(8) Consider hysteria as a cause of hyperventilation or apnoea and bear in mind the possibilities of a cerebrovascular accident or anaesthetic drug effect.
(9) Physiotherapy should also be requested.

Intermaxillary Fixation

(1) Give antiemetics. If the patient is not fully conscious, ask a trained attendant to watch over the patient and keep wirecutters to hand.

(2) You should rehearse the release of intermaxillary fixation with each new nursing attendant involved in that patient's care. Suction, light and oxygen should always be available during recovery.
(3) Warn the anaesthetist and arrange intensive care (if this is conventional with your unit). Use the tongue suture in the event of airway difficulties; sometimes firm pressure to advance the angle of the mandible will reopen the airway.

Acute Respiratory Obstruction

The patient may exhibit:
Cyanosis
Restlessness or struggling
Poor conscious level
Frustrated or accentuated respiratory efforts/noises.
Quickly see if you can ascertain the cause of obstruction and correct it, e.g. foreign body, denture, vomit, intermaxillary fixation. For this you will need an assistant, good light or a laryngoscope, suction, and the patient will need to be lying supine.

Attempt ventilation via oropharyngeal airway and Ambu-pack. If the patient's condition is deteriorating rapidly, then intubate the trachea urgently, and if this is not possible then carry out tracheostomy (see pp. 71–2). Once the airway is established, quickly reoxygenate.

FLUID REPLACEMENT

Consider the alternatives such as nasogastric feeding, encouraging oral fluids (see Chapter 19). The indications for intravenous infusion are:
(1) Urgent control of fluid, blood or certain constituents (electrolytes, glucose, plasma factors).
(2) Shock (traumatic/surgical following blood loss).
(3) Hypotension (dehydration or venous pooling, peripheral vasodilatation).
(4) Cachexia or anaemia (preoperative protein/calorie supplements, whole blood).
(5) The need to avoid oral contamination during healing.
(6) Inability to take oral fluids (disturbed consciousness or dysphagia).

Fluid Requirements

A healthy adult requires approximately 3 litres of fluid daily, e.g. 1 litre each of normal saline, 5% dextrose, Hartmann's solution. Patients with poor renal or cardiac function may require less. Vomiting, diarrhoea, drains or exudate from open or dressed wounds and regular aspiration, pyrexia and catabolic states all increase fluid requirements.

Older patients do not tolerate rapid infusion well. Children, of course, have modified fluid requirements. The clinical signs of fluid overload are a raised jugular venous pressure, dyspnoea, pitting oedema of the ankles or sacrum, coarse basal pulmonary crepitations.

Ideally monitor fluid replacement with a central venous pressure line, especially if large volumes or rapid replacement is required. If fluid overload occurs, sit the patient up, slow the infusion and give a rapid acting diuretic such as frusemide 40 mg.

Intravenous Materials

Crystalloids—(short lasting effect)
- Normal saline
- Dextrose (5%)
- Hartmann's solution

Colloids—(longer lasting effect, but take blood beforehand for crossmatching purposes)
- Dextran
- Haemaccel
- Intralipid }
- Vamin } intravenous nutrition
- Aminoplex }

Blood products
- Blood (whole/fresh/packed cells)
- Blood products (plasma, platelets, clotting factors, albumin)

Blood Transfusions

(1) Obtain specimens to test for haemoglobin, packed cell volume (PCV), urea and electrolytes and crossmatch.
(2) Blood is expensive and may be of limited availability.
(3) Never plan to use less than 2 units.

(4) Check all labels carefully on bottles and crossmatch requests, as mismatched transfusions are dangerous.
(5) Crossmatch electively as the urgent technique leaves less time for the laboratory to resolve incompatability.
(6) Tell the laboratory within 36 hours if crossmatched blood is not needed.
(7) Beware of transfusion overload, especially in the very young and the very old.

Transfusion Reaction

Haemolytic
Allergies and pyrogens
The effects of prolonged blood storage (hyperkalaemia, citrate toxicity)

Clinical signs

Shock, fever, rigor, loin pain, urticaria, tachycardia, haemoglobinuria.

Action

(1) Stop infusion.
(2) Replace the giving set (keep the old bag and giving set for laboratory analysis).
(3) Contact the haematologists.
(4) Commence intravenous infusion with sodium bicarbonate 4.2% and observe urine output carefully.
(5) Infuse approximately 50 ml of 25% mannitol over 2 hours check that the urine output is satisfactory.
(6) Infuse 1 g of hydrocortisone; frusemide 40 mg stat; chlorpheniramine maleate (up to 10 mg i.v.). Adrenaline may be required, control its dilution before infusion.

Chapter 5

Special Investigations and Use of the Laboratory

HAEMATOLOGICAL INVESTIGATIONS

Check with the laboratory regarding the amount of blood required for all haematological and biochemical tests. Use the correct specimen bottle (see Appendix D., pp. 201–2).

Virtually all haematological laboratories use automated counters to generate a haemoglobin value, a variety of red cell indices, a white count and in many cases a platelet count on routine samples. On review, further appropriate tests, such as B12, red cell folate, serum iron and total iron binding capacity may need to be performed.

Sore Mouth Investigations

These include a full blood count, blood film, ESR, serum ferritin, serum B12, serum and red blood cell folate. Where the findings indicate marrow pathology, a bone marrow aspirate may be appropriate after discussion with a haematologist.

Patients Undergoing Major Surgery

Perform a haematological screen checking haemoglobin, platelets, urea and electrolytes and a coagulation screen to establish a presurgical baseline and allow preoperative correction of any abnormalities revealed. Where malignant disease is present, request liver function tests.

Blood Replacement (see also Chapter 4)

Blood is available as whole blood or packed cells (if circulatory overload likely to be a problem). Do not order blood unless its use is likely. An alternative is to have the patient's blood grouped and the serum saved as this enables a fast supply if required. Postoperatively, where blood loss has occurred, haemoglobin is mandatory.

Routine Haemostatic Tests

Platelets

The normal range is 150–400 × 10^9/l. Generally if more than 40 × 10^9/l then spontaneous bleeding is uncommon whereas if less than 20 × 10^9/l, spontaneous bleeding is common.

Coagulation Screen

Prothrombin time (PT), thrombin time and kaolin cephalin time (KCT, PTT, PTTK) tests are used. Check with the haematology department to find the local normal ranges.

Prothrombin time

This tests the extrinsic blood coagulation system (I (fibrinogen), II, V, VII, X) and may be expressed as a prothrombin time or ratio. It is normal in haemophilia A and B but abnormal in patients with hepatic disease and those on oral anticoagulant therapy.

Kaolin cephalin time (KCT, PTT, PTTK)

This reflects the abnormalities in the intrinsic blood coagulation system (factor XII, Fletcher factor, high molecular weight kinogen, XI, IX, VIII, X, V, II and fibrinogen).

Thrombin time (TT)

This tests the terminal stages of the clotting pathways. The common causes of abnormalities are patients with low fibrinogen levels or inhibitors of thrombin, e.g. heparin, fibrin degradation products (FDPs) and dysfibrinogenaemia.

Patients on Anticoagulants

Patients are placed on anticoagulants following myocardial infarction, venous thrombosis and in some cases of valve abnormalities or replacement.

Heparin

Heparin may be given several ways:
(1) *Subcutaneous prophylactic heparin (minihep)*—With this regimen dental procedures should not be a problem.
(2) *Heparin by bolus*—Ideally should not be used in patients suspected of thrombosis. Consult haematologist prior to treatment.
(3) *Heparin by continuous infusion*—Therapeutic levels should be between 2–4 times the control KCT (PTT, PTTK).

Dental treatment can be carried out at the lower end of therapeutic range if necessary.

Warfarin or phenindione

Dosage is monitored by the prothrombin time (or prothrombin ratio) or by the commercial Thrombotest.
Prothrombin ratio:

$$\frac{\text{Patient's prothrombin time}}{\text{Normal prothrombin time}} \quad \text{(normal ratio is less than 1.3)}$$

The target range for anticoagulation is 2–4.5. Dental treatment should be carried out at the lower end of the therapeutic range (2). The higher the ratio the greater the risk of bleeding.
Thrombotest:
Normal—more than 70%
Therapeutic range 5–15%
Dental treatment at 15% level

Oral Surgery for the Anticoagulated Patient

Minor surgery of several teeth can be carried out at the lower end of the therapeutic range. Discuss with the haematologist/physician warfarin control prior to surgery. Do not arrange major surgery without specialist consultation.

Investigation of a Patient with a Suspected Bleeding Disorder

Ask specific questions on operations and complications. Bleeding can be spontaneous or delayed postinjury. Ask about site, extent, duration and frequency. Carry out a physical examination. Consider vascular defects, coagulation defects, platelet defects and associated conditions (anticoagulant therapy, hepatic disease, renal disease and drugs, such as aspirin, non-steroidal anti-inflammatory agents, broad spectrum antibiotics).

To investigate a bleeding disorder liaise with the haematologist, but basic blood investigations should include a full blood count with platelets and a clotting screen, a kaolin cephalin time to test the intrinsic clotting system, and a prothrombin time to test the extrinsic clotting system.

Haemophilia A and B would normally give a prolonged KCT, whereas liver-related abnormalities of the clotting pathway generally present with a prolonged prothrombin time. All patients found to have haemophilia or a platelet disorder are issued with a book detailing the disorder and the name of a haemophilia centre managing the day-to-day problems.

Summary of Investigations of a Patient with a Suspected Bleeding Disorder

Investigations

FBC
Platelets
Clotting screen
 KCT, PTT
 PT
 TT

Platelets

Normal haemostasis > 80 000
Bruising 20 000–80 000
Spontaneous haemorrhage < 20 000

Anticoagulation

Heparin prolongs PTT
Warfarin prolongs PT monitored by:
 Prothrombin time
 Prothrombin ratio
 Thrombotest

Minor surgery can be carried out without alteration of anticoagulation if:

PT is within normal therapeutic range (2–2.5 times normal)
Prothrombin ratio is at the lower end of the therapeutic range (2–4), e.g. 2 Thrombotest at 15% level.

Haemophilia A and B

Sex linked recessive (male affected, female carrier). Positive family history.
Haemophilia A, factor VIII deficient; haemophilia B, factor IX deficient.
Common sites of bleeding: gingiva, nose, joints, muscle.

Management of a Patient with a Known Bleeding Disorder

Platelet disorders

The most common abnormality of platelets likely to be encountered will be idiopathic thrombocytopenic purpura, where a platelet autoantibody destroys the platelets, rendering the patient thrombocytopenic.

Haemophilia

Mild—DDAVP (increases VIII activity)
Others—Factor VIII concentrates: cryoprecipitate, heat-treated freeze-dried (eliminates HTLVIII)

Half life VIII is 12 hours. For minor surgery the induction dose is 3000 units with 1000 units twice daily postoperatively. IU = activity in 1 ml normal plasma.

Oral surgery

All haemophiliacs should carry a book detailing the name of their haemophilia centre, factor levels, hepatitis status, the presence of inhibitors and other useful information.

For major surgery, factor replacement to give levels well within the normal range will be required.

The severity of the haemophilia will determine the nature of the factor replacement. Generally the severe haemophiliac will require factor concentrates or cryoprecipitates, whereas in the milder haemophiliacs DDAVP may be sufficient to raise the endogenous factor VIII level.

In von Willebrand's disease factor replacement with cryoprecipitate is usually required. These treatments are usually administered concurrently with an antifibrinolytic agent, such as tranexamic acid. Patients should be covered with an antibiotic.

The operative procedure and replacement therapy should be discussed well in advance with the haematologist.

Avoid intramuscular injections and inferior dental nerve injection. For infiltration of local anaesthetic use the interdental papilla. Use oral endotracheal intubation in preference to nasoendotracheal intubation where possible.

Disseminated intravascular coagulation (DIC)

In this disorder the balance between coagulation and fibrinolysis is out of order. Generalised intravascular fibrin production and thrombocytopenia may occur leading to a failure of haemostasis.

Precipitating factors are severe trauma, burns, incompatible transfusions, infections, obstetric complications, tumours, renal disease, liver disease, hypoxia and shock.

Investigations for suspected cases—Haemoglobin, blood film, platelet count, a full clotting screen including fibrin degradation products.

Management—Consult haematologist.

Sickle cell syndromes and sickle cell trait

This disorder affects many races, not just negroes. The heterozygous form is common and called sickle cell trait (Hb AS), whereas the homozygous form, sickle cell disease (Hb SS) is rarer. Other inherited haemoglobin abnormalities may also interact with the sickle gene to give a variety of other conditions collectively called the 'sickle cell syndromes'. Patients with sickle cell trait are not specifically at operative risk, but all the sickle cell syndromes may have sickling crises precipitated by a general anaesthetic.

All non-caucasians must be checked preoperatively to exclude the presence of sickle haemoglobin. The usual screening test is a rapidly available solubility test where the relative insolubility of reduced sickle haemoglobin allows for easy detection. When sickle haemoglobin is detected, a haemoglobin electrophoresis is essential to determine whether the patient has the trait or one of the sickle cell syndromes. If a sickle cell syndrome is discovered, the operative management should be discussed with the haematologist and anaesthetist presurgery.

Hepatitis

The most common causes are hepatitis A virus (HAV) and hepatitis B virus (HBV), but many other viruses may cause hepatitis, e.g. cytomegalovirus (CMV) and the Epstein-Barr virus (EBV).

HBV is spread parenterally and sexually; 5–10% of cases of HBV infection become carriers. Most carriers are symptomless, a proportion have chronic persistent hepatitis with a good prognosis or chronic active hepatitis with a poorer prognosis leading to cirrhosis. Patients with a past history of hepatitis and high risk groups (i.v. drug abusers, male homosexuals, patients receiving blood products, e.g. haemophiliacs, immunosuppressed, dialysed patients, high risk ethnic groups, e.g. Africans and Chinese) should be screened for serum markers of HBV.

Serum markers of HBV

Markers appear 4–15 weeks post-contact. Symptoms appear 4–6 weeks later. Infection markers remain for 6–16 weeks, a continued presence after 6 months suggests a *carrier*. HBs Ag appears first, followed by HBc Ag. In most cases HBc begins to disappear and is replaced by anti HBc. The last overt infection marker to go is HBs Ag and this is replaced within 2–3 weeks in 90% of cases by anti HBs. There is a 'window' between the disappearance of HBs Ag and the appearance of anti HBs during which the only markers present are anti core markers.

In the carrier HBs Ag is detectable potentially for life. In approximately one-third of all carriers, HBe is found and indicates high infectivity; the remainder of the HBs carriers have anti HBc indicative of a much reduced level of infectivity. A small proportion of all carriers (less than 18%) have anti core (anti HBc) as the only marker.

Management of suspected patients

Send serum to determine HBs Ag status; generally a result is obtained within 24 hours. If negative treat as normal, if positive take special precautions.

Use disposable instruments where possible, treat patients at the end of the day, use adequate protection, such as gowns, masks, gloves, glasses. Avoid aerosol-producing instruments. Non-disposables can be autoclaved, placed in hot air ovens or immersed in 2% glutaraldehyde (Cidex) for several hours. All working surfaces must be disinfected with Cidex.

Prevention

Vaccine to HBV is now available as a three-dose course; 90% of vaccinees become immune to HBV. Where inoculation occurs from a suspected carrier, wash the puncture site with water, take a sample of the patient's blood to determine infectivity and contact the virologist for immunoglobulin administration.

AIDS (acquired immune deficiency syndrome)

This is the name given to a symptom complex of health problems. There is a breakdown of the body's immune system, the main defect being in cell mediated immunity. Patients become vulnerable to opportunistic infections and a 90% 2 year fatality rate has been reported.

The causative virus is believed to be an RNA retrovirus, human T cell lymphotrophic virus (HTLV-III) or lymphadenopathy associated virus (LAV). The majority of patients affected are male homosexuals or bisexuals, but other groups affected include intravenous drug abusers, haemophiliacs and recipients of infected blood products. Infectivity is low, spread is much the same as hepatitis B virus (HBV). Incubation periods are long and can be years.

Presentation is varied, sufferers may present with lymphadenopathy, fatigue, opportunistic infections, especially candidiasis, toxoplasma, herpes virus infections and cytomegalovirus. There are two rare diseases associated with AIDS, Kaposi's sarcoma and *Pneumocystis carinii* pneumonia.

Patients with clinical AIDS should be treated in the same way as patients who have HBV, using the same precautions.

MICROBIOLOGY

All specimens go into sterile containers prior to antibiotic administration if possible. The best specimen is pus, sent in a universal container, aspirated into a syringe or onto an applicator stick in a sterile tube which may contain a transport medium. Label all specimens, give adequate history indicating if the patient is on antibiotics, otherwise the laboratory will not know which cultures to perform or how to interpret the results. Give the date and time of collection.

Blood Culture

Take this from any patient with suspected systemic infection (fever, shock, rigors, general malaise). Discuss the patient with the microbiologist at an early stage.

Technique

(1) Reduce skin contamination at venepuncture site, use 70% alcohol.
(2) Withdraw 10 ml of blood and divide between two broths (aerobic and anaerobic incubation).
(3) Swab top of culture bottles, change needle prior to inoculating cultures.
(4) Only use *fresh* media, send to laboratory as soon as possible with clinical information and antibiotic regimen if any. Results are usually available in 1–3 days.

Gram Stain

Gram-positive organisms appear blue as they retain the dye complex of methyl violet and iodine and are not discoloured after the decolorisation procedure. Gram-negative organisms appear red because of counter stain used after decolorisation. Pus cells are also shown, and the results are available within half an hour of receipt of specimen in the laboratory.

Plating a Swab

This is usually carried out by a laboratory technician, a variety of selective media and cultural conditions can be used depending on clinical details. Sensitivity results can be obtained by placing antibiotic-impregnated discs onto inoculated agar. Results are available within 24–48 hours. *Note* cultures from oropharynx grow many commensal bacteria of doubtful pathogenic significance.

Virology

When serum specimens are taken remember to take the acute phase serum immediately and the convalescent serum 2 weeks later to compare the antibody titre. Certain virus infections, e.g. herpes, can be diagnosed directly by electron microscopy. Contact the department of virology to see if this service exists.

RADIOLOGICAL INVESTIGATIONS

Intraoral Radiographs

(1) Dental caries—Periapical radiographs, bite-wing radiographs (show interdental area).
(2) Wisdom teeth—Dental X-rays, OPG, right and left lateral oblique.
(3) Canines—Parallax views using either periapicals or maxillary occlusals, vertex occlusal, true lateral skull, PA jaws.
(4) Calculi—Can be shown in the submandibular or parotid ducts initially by plain film if they are radio-opaque. Dental film over the calculi, mandibular true occlusal, mandibular oblique occlusal, OPG and sialography.

Extraoral Radiographs (Facial Bones)

The radiographs commonly used are occipitomental 15°, 30° and 45°, true lateral, PA mandible, right and left lateral obliques, OPG, submentovertex. Occipitomentals (15°) demonstrate the frontal sinus, maxillary sinus, nasal bones and antral fluid levels. Views of 30° are ideal for fractures and middle-third of the face showing the orbital rims, the orbital floor, the zygomatic arches and the malar complexes. Submentovertex views show the zygomatic arches, the base of the skull and the nasopharynx.

Temporomandibular Joint Views

High OPG open and closed, lateral transcranio-oblique shows condylar head plus joint space; reverse Towne's (shows condyle and rami, for fractures of condylar neck); transpharyngeal shows condylar head but not the joint space; transorbital (Zimmer's view) for AP view of condylar head.

Cephalometrics

Used for orthodontics and orthognathic surgery, X-rays are nearly parallel (giving minimal distortion)—teeth in occlusion, lips at rest. Lateral and postero-anterior views (for facial asymmetries).

Tomography

Coronal or sagittal, only desired plane in focus, used for blow-out fractures, temporomandibular joints, etc.

Sialography

Commonly performed on parotid and submandibular glands to show ductal structure. Used to demonstrate stones, strictures, space occupying lesions within glands.

CT Scan (Computer Tomography)

These are X-ray scans. The electronic detectors pick up X-rays and store information on floppy discs which can be demonstrated on a visual display unit. Both hard and soft tissues are demonstrated. These are ideal to show extent of tumours in head and neck region.

Isotope Scanning

Technetium 99^{m} pertechnetate is avidly taken up by all salivary tissue hence its use in salivary gland scanning. There is increased uptake in Warthin's tumour, but it is not generally helpful however in illustrating salivary gland tumours.

Isotope bone imaging is used for investigations for primary and secondary malignant disease to identify bone metastasis. Areas of increased bone metabolism show increased uptake of radio-isotope which is injected intravenously and emits gamma rays detected by a gamma camera. Increased areas of uptake show up as dark areas on the scan.

Radiological Requests for Maxillofacial Trauma

The following are necessary: cranial views to exclude skull fracture, posterior, anterior and lateral skull views, occipitomental 15°, 30° and 45° to show facial bones and the middle-third of the facial skeleton maxillary occlusal to detect palatal fractures, OPG to show mandible and dentition, and dental films to demonstrate individual tooth fracture.

Mandibular Fractures

The following are necessary: OPG or right and left lateral obliques, PA mandible, mandibular occlusal, dental films. To show condyle OPG, reverse Towne's, transpharyngeal views are used as required.

Note If teeth and fillings are missing and unaccounted for, a chest X-ray is mandatory. If patients are involved in severe trauma, other bony injuries may be present and these should be excluded by taking the appropriate X-rays.

PHOTOGRAPHY

Photography is used to record lesions and their progression. Where lesions are photographed, place a centimetre rule adjacent to show the size. It is particularly useful in trauma cases where litigation may follow, and especially in orthognathic surgery cases where pre- and post-treatment photographs form part of the case notes.

Orthognathic Photography

This should be done both preoperatively and postoperatively. Request colour slides and black and white prints. Photographs should include full face and profile in 1:1 ratio. These can be used in conjunction with lateral cephalogram for profile prediction. Pin the hair off the face. Photographs required: teeth in occlusion, anterior view and 45° views from the right and left.

MAXILLOFACIAL LABORATORY AIDS

Become acquainted with procedures and techniques in the laboratory. Consider asking the advice of the technicians as they may have knowledge of the consultant's preferences.

Laboratory Cards

Give clear concise instructions, write in ink, date, sign and indicate consultant in charge. Use one laboratory card only. Inform the technician of any changes required from the original prescription. Draw diagrams to indicate design, making special mention of the position of fractures, teeth to be extracted, crown and bridgework. Indicate the position of proposed wiring. It is advisable to have loops for circumzygomatic wires in maxillary splints even if they are not used.

Impressions

Good technical work needs good impressions (remove all debris from teeth beforehand). Where tooth grinding is necessary, do so prior to impression. For accurate bite registration use wax on which the occlusal plane and centre line is marked. Have impressions cast as soon as possible.

Fractures

Laboratory facilities are necessary for Gunning splints, custom-made arch bars and cast cap splints. In edentulous fractures give the technician the patient's old dentures, fractured or not. These can be used to pour models enabling construction of Gunning splints with correct occlusion and vertical dimension. *Do not* use the patient's dentures as Gunning splints as the unit may be responsible for providing new ones.

Special Requirements

(1) Gutta percha lining.
(2) Grooves for transalveolar and circum-mandibular wires.
(3) Loops for circumzygomatic wires.

Splints

Design splints properly, inform the technician of the proposed surgery and operation date, and discuss special requirements with the technician.

Splint cementation

(1) Try the splints prior to cementation.
(2) Block all holes with wax before cementation.

(3) Check the projection rod does not interfere with soft tissues.
(4) Mix black copper cement properly—it is advisable to use gloves.
(5) Remove excess cement with cotton wool soaked in sodium bicarbonate solution.
(6) Warn patients of nausea postcementation, prevent electrolytic ulcers from forming by placing wax on the localisation plates.

Splint removal

(1) Allow sufficient time (approximately 1 hour) for splint removal.
(2) Use splint removal forceps or old extraction forceps.
(3) Place one blade on the occlusal surface, the other beneath the cleat and gently squeeze to break the cement seal. Do this in several places. Beware of crowned teeth.
(4) Remove all cement and advise the patient on oral hygiene technique. Take postoperative photographs of the occlusion in 1–2 weeks when all the cement is off the teeth and the mucosa is healing.

Osteotomy Cases

Take your work-box to the theatre, it should include pre- and postoperative models, wafers and accessories, e.g. projection rods, marked locking plates, marked screws. These are usually placed on a waxed sheet which can be given to the theatre sister to sterilise prior to the operation. It is also advisable to have spare screws which have been tested to check that they fit locking plates.

Eyelet Wires

The house surgeon is responsible for an adequate supply of all wires to the theatre. Use 0.5 stainless steel wire, prestretch by 10% (3 m length stretched to 3.3 m), cut off 15 cm at either end because of the work hardening. Eyelets are made using 15 cm lengths wound around a burr shank and twisted $2\frac{1}{2}$ times. They are cut to equal lengths and placed on a safety pin for sterilisation.

Obturators

Plan surgery with obturators in mind. Provide adequate retention, make a temporary appliance to prevent tissue shrinkage. Obturators can be complicated and difficult, so see the patient jointly with the technician. Impressions for the special tray are taken in alginate, avoid flow into the nasal cavities and the breakage of alginate on removal. Use either alginate or a rubber base material, then build up the bung in wax.

Obturators are time consuming and sufficient time and patience must be allocated. Minutes spent carefully in the impression stage can save hours of frustration later. The patient must be given regular appointments at weekly intervals. Make obturators as light as possible, considering the use of sectional obturators with Molloplast for retention and ease of placement.

Chapter 6

Common Practical Procedures

VENEPUNCTURE

(1) Reassure the patient and explain the procedure.
(2) Clean the skin using 5% chlorhexidine and 70% alcohol or Mediswab.
(3) Obtain sufficient blood for the investigations required. If a large volume of blood is required place an in-dwelling cannula.

Sites of Puncture

These are commonly antecubital fossa or dorsum of the hand, occasionally the forearm, and, in the last resort, the femoral vein (Fig. 6.1).

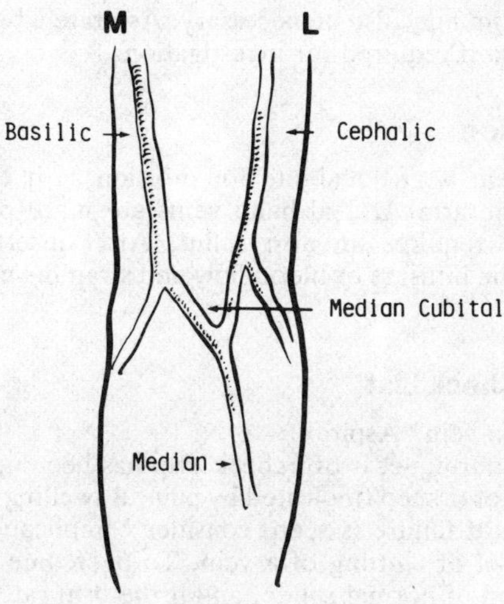

Fig. 6.1 Cubital fossa and veins

Technique

(1) Apply a tourniquet proximal to the site of puncture, avoid arterial obstruction, tap overlying skin, fix vein by stretching.
(2) Insert needle with bevel up applying gentle suction.
(3) Withdraw blood slowly to prevent haemolysis then release tourniquet, remove the needle and apply pressure to avoid haematoma.

INTRAVENOUS INFUSION

Prevent bacteraemia by employing a strict aseptic technique, shave any hair from the patient's arm first.

Equipment

Use a single chamber infusion-giving set for infusions of non-blood products and a double chamber set for blood transfusion. (Run normal saline into the giving set prior to commencing a blood transfusion.) Use a large bore intravenous cannula (16 gauge or larger). Always have a second ready at the time of setting up a drip. Adhesive strips are needed to secure the cannula in position, a bandage and splint may also be necessary. Aspirate a blood sample from the cannula if required for investigations.

Sites of Infusion

The cephalic vein is an ideal site for infusion as it enables free movement of the arm. Dorsal hand veins are more painful. The antecubital site requires an arm splint. After insertion of the cannula check the infusate or blood flow and strap the cannula with adhesive tape.

Drip Failure Check List

(1) Is cannula in vein? Aspirate.
(2) Check the tourniquet is off, check drip has been opened fully, check drip has not tissued (indicated by painful swelling at the site).
(3) If no cause of failure is seen, consider complications such as spasm of a vessel or clotting of a vein. To overcome this, gently syringe with 5 ml of normal saline, and if the drip rate is too slow raise the height of the drip stand.

CENTRAL VENOUS PRESSURE MEASUREMENT (RIGHT ATRIAL PRESSURE)

This is used as an index of effective circulating blood volume and is used in cases of replacement of large volumes of fluid when over- or undertransfusion can be detected quickly. Where signs of overload, e.g. raised jugular venous pressure (JVP), crepitations at lung bases and oedema occur these correspond to a raised central venous pressure (CVP) measurement.

The CVP measurement is an indication of the pressure in the right atrium and the great intrathoracic veins. To measure CVP the catheter is inserted into the right atrium via a forearm vein, subclavian or internal jugular vein.

The normal CVP lies between 5–10 cmH_2O—a reading less than 5 cmH_2O indicates hypovolaemia.

ARTERIAL BLOOD GASES

These are commonly used to measure the pH, Pao_2 and $Paco_2$ of blood (*see* Appendix C., p. 200). They indicate the extent of respiratory or metabolic acidosis and alkalosis and are used to monitor the ventilated patient.

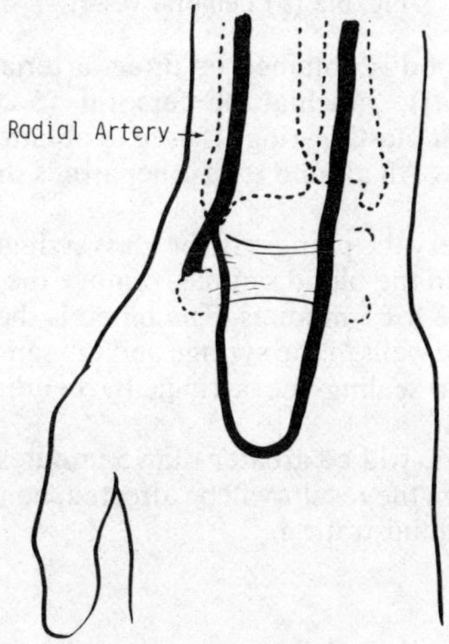

Fig. 6.2 (*a*) Radial artery puncture site.

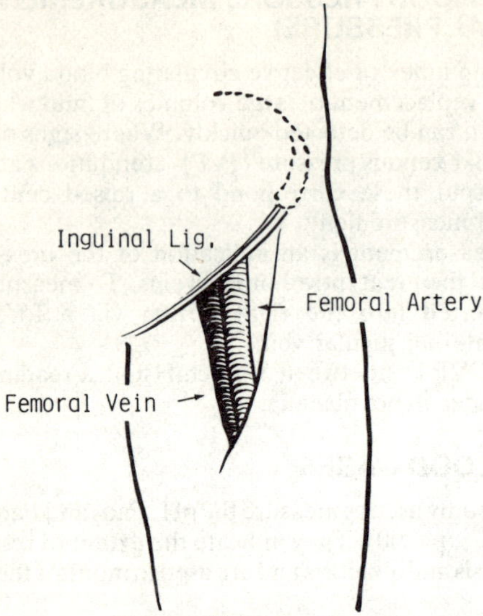

Fig. 6.2 (*b*) Femoral vessels.

A sample of blood is obtained by direct arterial puncture, using radial (Fig. 6.2(*a*)), brachial or femoral (6.2(*b*)) arteries. A heparinised glass or plastic syringe is used to obtain a blood sample, 5 ml being sufficient. All air and excess heparin is then expelled from the syringe.

When in the artery the plunger in the glass syringe will rise because of pressure. Obtain the blood sample, remove the needle and apply pressure to the site for 5 minutes. The blood is then mixed with the heparin on the side walls of the syringe and the sample sent for blood gas analysis, after sealing the syringe by bending the needle or capping.

If the transit time will be greater than 5 minutes, pack in ice. If a patient is on oxygen the results will be affected, hence write down the rate of oxygen administration.

Results

(1) *pH*—Normal range pH 7.36–7.42. In compensated acidosis or alkalosis the pH stays within the normal range.

(2) *Standard bicarbonate*—Normal range 21–26 mmol/l. Plasma bicarbonate *alone* does not indicate whether acidosis or alkalosis is present. It must be known if the primary disturbances are respiratory in origin.
(3) *Blood* $Paco_2$—Normal range 34–46 mmHg (4.5–6.0 kPa)
$Paco_2$ is increased with hypoventilation (respiratory acidosis).
$Paco_2$ is decreased with hyperventilation (respiratory alkalosis).
(4) *Blood* Pao_2—Normal range 80–100 mmHg (10.6–13.2 kPa)
Pao_2 is increased by oxygen administration.
(5) *Base excess*—Measured as −2 + 2 mmol/l, a measure of surplus acid or base in the blood. In metabolic acidosis (for example diabetic ketoacidosis) there is a base deficit. In metabolic alkalosis (for example vomiting) there is a base excess.

INTRAMUSCULAR INJECTIONS

Common sites for intramuscular injection are the deltoid area, anterior thigh and buttock. Injections in the buttock can injure the sciatic nerve, therefore use a 'safe area' such as the upper outer quadrant which avoids sciatic nerve injury (Fig. 6.3, p. 68).

Place the outstretched hand with thumb and thenar eminence along the iliac crest, the thumb tip touching the anterior superior iliac spine. The area beneath the hand is 'safe'. Stretch the skin, cleanse, and insert the needle by giving a sharp quick jab at 90° to the skin, aspirate and inject slowly, withdraw the needle quickly and massage the site.

SUBCUTANEOUS INJECTIONS

For subcutaneous injection, e.g. insulin injection, use the outer aspect of the upper arm, outer aspect of upper thigh, and skin of the abdominal wall. These areas can be used for small volume (1–2 ml) administration.

URINE COLLECTION

This is usually a nursing procedure. A mid-stream specimen of urine (MSU) is obtained for bacterial examination, and the specimen should be transported to the laboratory within 1 hour or refrigerated at 4° C.

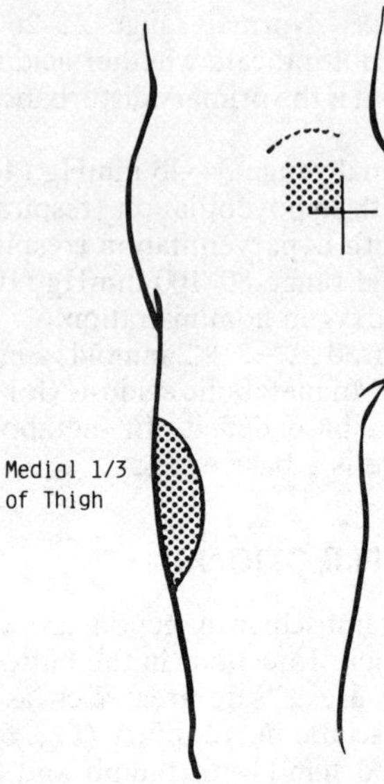

Fig. 6.3 Site for intramuscular injections.

In the *male* retract the foreskin, clean the glans, collect the urine after the urethral contents are clear, catch the specimen in mid-stream into a sterile bottle. An early morning specimen should be obtained.

In the *female* specimens are preferably obtained by female staff.

Bladder Catheterisation

A Foley catheter is most commonly used.

Male

(1) Use an aseptic technique—Mask, gloves, gown.
(2) Clean the pubic area, drape the patient.
(3) Clean the penis with 1% chlorhexidine solution. Retract the foreskin and clean the glans.
(4) Use 1% lignocaine gel 10 ml to anaesthetise the urethra using a special nozzle and a penile clamp.

(5) Allow 2 minutes for the urethra to become anaesthetised. Lubricate the catheter, use 18 G (have 16 G and 14 G ready as well). Have the receptacle ready for the collection of urine.
(6) Hold the penis in the left hand, remove the perforated end of the sterile packaging of the catheter and gently introduce the catheter into the urethra.
(7) Start with an 18 G Foley catheter and when urine flow is established fill the balloon with the correct amount of normal saline (stated on the catheter).
(8) Send the specimen obtained for culture and sensitivity tests. Spigot catheter or attach to collecting bag.

Female

Catheterisation should preferably be delegated to female staff.

NASOGASTRIC INTUBATION

Ryle's Tube

(1) Sit patient up, inspect nasal airway for deformity.
(2) Lubricate the chilled tube, pass the tube via the nose into the nasopharynx and ask the patient to take deep breaths.
(3) Ask the patient to take a full mouth of water and while advancing the tube ask the patient to swallow.
(4) The tube should pass into the oesophagus and then to the stomach. However, if the patient coughs it may have entered the larynx in which case withdraw the tube, reposition the patient's head and reinsert.
(5) Confirm the position of tube by aspiration. Place the aspirate on litmus paper; if the tube is in the stomach blue litmus paper turns red because of acid reaction.
(6) The position of the tube is checked by blowing a syringe full of air into the stomach and auscultating. If the tube is in the correct position tape the tube to nose and then spigot.

Minibore Tube

Nasogastric intubation of this tube is similar to the above procedure.
(1) Lubricate stylet with KY jelly to overcome difficulty in later removal when in position.

(2) Avoid forceful insertion.
(3) Check tube position by auscultation on syringing of air; administer a minimal volume normal saline down the tube noting cough reflex indicating incorrect position.
(4) Finally and most importantly check with a chest X-ray to indicate correct position prior to commencing feed which should be sterile clear fluids initially.

ENDOTRACHEAL INTUBATION

Requirements:
Laryngoscope
Endotracheal tube
Inflation bag
(1) Place the patient in the supine position.
(2) Stand behind the patient and extend the neck.
(3) Insert the laryngoscope, avoiding damage to the anterior teeth, (an acrylic or gutta percha splint may be used to safeguard crowns and bridges).
(4) Pull the tongue forward with the laryngoscope, visualise vocal cords. Pressure on cricoid may also be of value.
(5) Insert the lubricated endotracheal tube, through the cords into the trachea, then inflate the cuff.
(6) Connect the tube to the inflation bag and check to ensure expansion of the lungs.

CRICOTHYROTOMY (LARYNGOSTOMY)

For acute laryngeal obstruction where an endotracheal tube cannot be passed cricothyrotomy can be used as a temporary life saving procedure and is far safer to perform than an emergency tracheostomy by inexperienced hands (Fig. 6.4).

Method

A wide bore needle 12–14 gauge is inserted into the space between the thyroid cartilage and the cricoid piercing the cricothyroid membrane. This needle is connected to a high pressure oxygen jet.

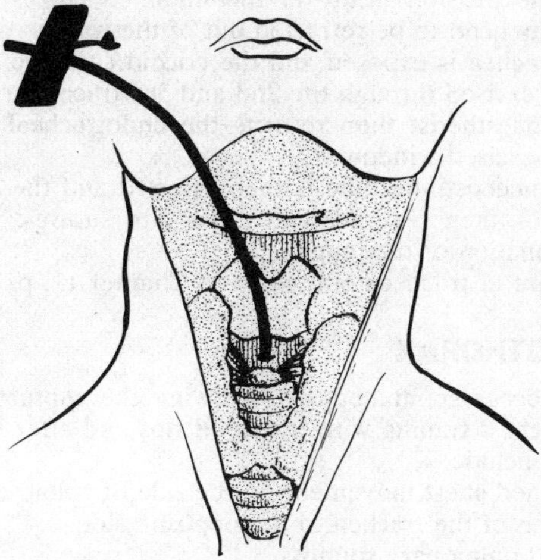

Fig. 6.4 Cricothyrotomy.

TRACHEOSTOMY

This is normally an elective procedure carried out in theatre under a general anaesthetic with an endotracheal tube *in situ*. Obtain consent prior to operation and allay the patient's fears explaining to him that he will not be able to speak afterwards.

Requirements:

Standard tracheostomy set (always check the compatibility of all fittings).

Average tracheostomy tube, males 24–42; females 33–36 French gauge.

Method

(1) The patient's neck is extended with a sandbag placed under the shoulders.

(2) Mark the suprasternal notch and cricoid cartilage, the skin is then infiltrated with a vasoconstrictor. A horizontal skin incision is made midway between these landmarks.

(3) Blunt dissection is carried out through the strap muscles while

keeping the incision firmly in the midline. The isthmus of the thyroid may need to be retracted out of the way.
(4) The trachea is exposed and the cricoid cartilage identified. A window is excised through the 2nd and 3rd tracheal rings.
(5) The anaesthetist then retracts the endotracheal tube to just above the excised window.
(6) The tracheostomy tube is then inserted and the cuff inflated. The tube is then secured with tapes and sutures. Check for a uniform inflation of the lungs.
(7) For care of tracheostomy refer to Chapter 11, p. 117.

PNEUMOTHORAX

This can occur spontaneously following the rupture of a bulla, following chest trauma with fractured ribs and after rib resection. The signs include:

Diminished chest movement on the side of collapse.
Deviation of the trachea to the opposite side.
Reduced pulmonary sounds.
Hyper-resonance to percussion.
Observe collapsed lung edge on X-ray.

This condition is treated by the insertion of a chest drain.

Insertion of Chest Drain

Check the chest X-ray and identify the side to be drained. The following equipment is required: local anaesthetic, heavy suture 2.0 silk, needle holders, toothed forceps, trocar and catheter, heavy clamp and an underwater seal.

Method

(1) Observe full sterile procedure.
(2) The tube is inserted in the second intercostal space lateral to the mid-clavicular line or preferably the 4th or 5th intercostal space in the mid-axillary line.
(3) The skin is infiltrated with local anaesthetic.
(4) The trocar and catheter are then inserted into the pleural space, their passage aided by cutting skin with the scalpel.
(5) Insertion requires considerable force, the left hand is placed on the trocar and catheter 5 cm from the tip to act as a stop. Keep as close to the lower rib as possible to avoid intercostal vessels.

(6) The resistance on the trocar and catheter disappears as the pleural space is entered, the catheter is then pushed off the trocar and the tube is clamped as it is connected to an underwater seal drain.
(7) The clamp is then released. Check that air is escaping and fluid in the tube oscillates with respiration.
(8) A purse string suture of non-absorbable material is inserted around the tube such that it can be tied when the drain is finally removed.
(9) The drain is sutured to the skin and fixed with adhesive tape.
(10) X-ray and check that the lung has expanded.
(11) The drain is clamped after 24 hours.
(12) Check that there is no recurrent pneumothorax. If the X-ray shows full expansion the drain can be removed after asking patient to make deep inspiratory effort at the time of removal.
(13) The skin is then closed with the previously placed purse string suture and a dressing is applied.

BIOPSY

Principles

Excisional biopsy is performed if the lesion is less than 1 cm in diameter, incisional biopsy is employed for larger lesions. The most suspicious area is then chosen (the toluidine dye test may help—*see* Appendix G., p. 204) and the specimen orientated with sutures. Serial (geographic) biopsies may need to be performed. The pathologist must be given adequate patient history and measurements of the lesion. Draw diagrams with dimensions giving clinical details.

Types of Biopsy

The following are used: incisional, excisional, aspiration, punch, bone drill, exfoliative cytology. All biopsies must be of an adequate size and depth and have a margin of normal tissue. Wedge excisions are easier to close, the incision being kept parallel to important structures, such as nerves and vessels.

Handling the Specimen

(1) Avoid trauma an orientation suture should be placed in the specimen, then fix immediately in 10% formalin.

(2) Label all bottles carefully.
(3) If malignancy is suspected, mark 'urgent' and contact the pathologist.
(4) Make sure the histology report is seen by the clinician and placed in the patient's notes.
(5) Organise further treatment if necessary.

ELECTROCARDIOGRAPH (ECG)

This provides an electrical tracing of the heart. It is mandatory for all patients with a history or suspected history of cardiac disease.

Procedure

(1) Attach the electrodes with electrode jelly to hairless areas of the patient's limbs, e.g. inner forearm and outer aspects of legs.
(2) Attach the leads labelled as:

LA left arm	LF left foot
RA right arm	RF right foot

Check that all the connections are tight.
(3) Make sure that the patient is warm and relaxed.
(4) Standardise the recording so that one mV causes a deflection of 10 mm. Run a 6 cm of record for each lead.
(5) Between leads wait for the stylus to return to the baseline and alter the leads with the selector switch labelling each strip, e.g. I, II, aVF, etc.

Chest Leads

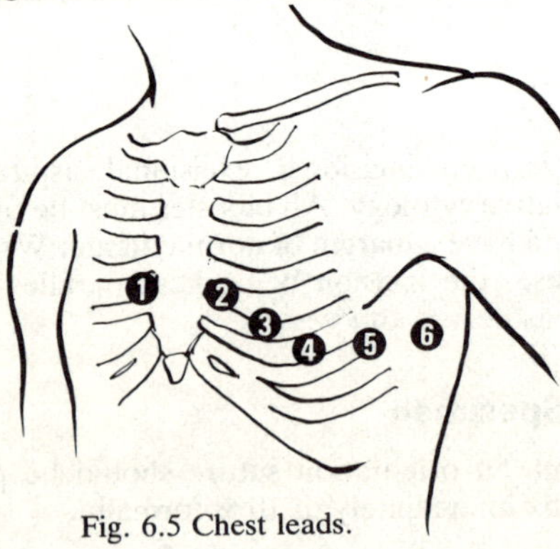

Fig. 6.5 Chest leads.

Note that:

V1 is the 4th intercostal space on the right side of the sternum
V2 is the 4th intercostal space on the left side of the sternum
V3 is midway between V2 and V4
V4 is the 5th intercostal space, mid clavicular line
V5 is anterior axillary line AAL level with V4
V6 mid axillary line level with V5

The first intercostal space is just above the sternal angle. The second intercostal space is just below the sternal angle.

OXYGEN ADMINISTRATION

Oxygen must be available in every clinical facility. It is used for the patient who has collapsed, is cyanosed, has had a cardiac arrest, has respiratory distress and in patients with angina-like chest pain.

Its administration is used to prevent tissue hypoxia and hypercapnia. Oxygen should be given in a sufficient concentration to raise the Pao_2 to at least 40 mmHg and higher. Beware of patients with chronic bronchitis and a raised $Paco_2$ as they rely on a fall in Pao_2 to stimulate respiration (hypoxic drive). A sudden rise in Pao_2 which reduces their hypoxic drive and depresses ventilation can be *extremely dangerous*.

Routinely 24% oxygen is firstly administered by Ventimask or nasal catheter. Masks allowing concentrations of 24%, 26%, 28%, 30%, 35%, 40% and 50% are all available. Directions for their administration are printed on packaging supplied with the mask.

BLOOD PRESSURE

(1) Position the patient at rest, with the arm resting at heart level.
(2) Place the cuff around the upper arm and while feeling the radial artery, inflate the cuff to 30 mm above loss of pulsation.
(3) The area over the brachial artery is then auscultated and the cuff slowly deflated.

(4) Systolic pressure is measured as that pressure which coincides with return of sound.
(5) As deflation continues sounds become muffled. The point at which sound disappears is diastolic pressure.
(6) Blood pressure is expressed as systolic pressure/diastolic pressure, e.g. 120/80 mmHg.

Chapter 7

Dentoalveolar Surgery

This can be carried out in either the surgery or the operating theatre. The type and extent of surgery depends on the result of presurgical assessment. One must take into account the patient's cooperation (local anaesthesia/local anaesthesia plus sedation/ general anaesthesia), medical contraindications, the extent of surgery and degree of difficulty. All surgery should, of course, be carried out under sterile conditions with the provision of a good light, suction, instrumentation and adequate assistance.

PRINCIPLES OF SURGERY

Know the *anatomy* of the region, proximity of nerves and blood vessels, density of bone, proximity to floor of nose and maxillary antrum.

Ensure adequate exposure of operating site. Have well designed flaps (large flaps are better than small), with suture lines over bone. Provide adequate analgesia, antibiotics (if required; *see* Chapter 3 and British National Formulary) and follow-up care.

ASSESSMENT

Anatomy

Inferior Dental Nerve

If there is risk of damage warn the patient. The nerve emerges as the mental nerve in the region of $\overline{54|45}$, take care in flap design, look for the emergence of the mental nerve and protect it.

Lingual Nerve

This is in intimate contact with periosteum in the third molar region; protect it with an instrument, e.g. Howarth periosteal elevator or Rowe lingual nerve retractor, to prevent damage with a chisel or burr. Do not use excessive retraction force on lingual tissues for fear of damage to this nerve.

Blood Vessels

The facial artery and a vein lie in the soft tissues opposite the $\overline{7|7}$. The long buccal artery lies in the cheek in the $\overline{8|8}$ area.

Bone

The lingual plate is thin in the $\overline{8|8}$ area. The buccal bone is thick. The maxillary tuberosity is often weak because of the size of the antrum. The maxillary antrum is in close association with the apices of the upper molar teeth, hence the likelihood of an oroantral fistula must be considered following extraction. In the maxilla the buccal bone is generally thinnest. Remember, the apices of the upper anterior teeth are often found near the floor of the nose; during operation, the nasal cavity, lined with mucosa, may be mistaken for an apical cyst.

RADIOGRAPHS

An OPG is a good screening radiograph. Dental periapical films, however, show greater detail. Radiographs are used to assess proximity of teeth to vital structures, carious involvement of teeth, presence of teeth, roots, cysts and bone density. The size, shape, position of roots and vitality (? root filled) should be assessed. Radiographs help anticipate problems such as root fracture, bone fracture, sinus involvement, and prior warning may reduce complications by planned flap elevation, bone removal and tooth sectioning.

GENERAL PROCEDURE

(1) Become acquainted with instruments available in the unit.
(2) Set up the instruments and materials in order of usage prior to surgery, e.g. local anaesthetic, retractor, scalpel. This eliminates missing essential items.

(3) Reassure the patient, check comfort of patient and operator, lubricate lips, avoid damage to soft tissue and adjoining teeth.
(4) Watch for overheating of a hand-piece; this is often prevented by the use of sharp burrs.
(5) In removing teeth use *controlled* force. If there is no movement of the tooth do not struggle with extraction but consider tooth division, or surgical removal, as this minimises discomfort and postoperative complications.

MUCOPERIOSTEAL FLAPS

Use as often as required to give access to bone, teeth and roots.

Principles

(1) Raise a good sized flap for access (a broad base improves blood supply) to allow an adequate margin of bone for repositioning.
(2) Cut through mucoperiosteum onto bone (facilitates the raising of a good flap) remembering local anatomy.
(3) Include interdental papillae in the flap (do not split the papillae).
(4) All cuts must be controlled, avoiding extension lingually in the retromolar area (lingual nerve), and special care should be taken with vertical cuts in the $\overline{54|55}$ area (mental nerve).
(5) Cut at right angles to the mucosa, cut in the depth of the gingival sulcus, extending to crestal bone, avoiding damage to interdental papillae.
(6) Raise mucoperiosteum cleanly with a periosteal elevator and retract gently.
(7) Remove bone and roots with sharp instruments and burrs using normal saline as a coolant and irrigant.

Wound Closure

(1) Debride and irrigate the wound.
(2) Replace tissue in original position using sutures of choice (usually 3/0 silk, 4/0 catgut).
(3) Avoid suturing a flap which is under tension, keeping sutures away from the edge of the flap.
(4) Intraoral sutures are left approximately 5 days.

MINOR ORAL SURGICAL PROCEDURES

Removal of roots
Removal of isolated upper molar teeth
Removal of third molars
Removal of unerupted canines
Apicectomy
Fraenectomy

Removal of Roots

(1) Use root forceps, elevators or probes.
(2) If the root is large and covered by mucosa and bone, raise a periosteal flap, remove bone and elevate root. If the apical root fragment is *in situ* and close to the inferior dental canal or antrum, consider leaving it as an attempt at removal may cause damage.
(3) Inform the patient of the presence of the root and make an entry in the notes.
(4) Multirooted teeth are large, divergent and difficult to remove and should be sectioned. This may require buccal flap and bone removal. After sectioning, remove roots separately with forceps or elevators.

Removal of Isolated Upper Molar Teeth

(1) Take care, check X-ray as tuberosity may be pneumatised and may fracture on extraction.
(2) Where pneumatised remove a tooth surgically to avoid fracturing tuberosity.
(3) Where tuberosity fractures occur raise a mucoperiosteal flap, free soft tissues, remove bone and close with mattress sutures to evert the edges. Leave sutures *in situ* for 10 days.

Removal of Third Molars (Mandibular)

Indications

Pericoronitis
Caries
Erosion of second molars

Clinical evaluation

(1) Assess with care.
(2) X-rays are essential to determine the degree of difficulty and suitability for removal in the dental chair.
(3) Consider access, position and depth, relationship to the ramus, second molar and inferior dental canal.
(4) Warn the patient of possible complications, if any.
(5) The ideal age for removal of the third molars is 16–21 years, as bone is elastic and there are fewer complications.

Generally

Beware of distoangular impactions. Look at the root pattern, crown shape, bone texture, thickness of interdental bone between the second and third molars, proximity to the inferior dental canal, with due regard to restorations in the adjoining teeth, if any.

Warn patients of probable complications beforehand.

Unerupted Canines

(1) Use periapical or occlusal radiographs with parallax views (if tooth moves in direction of X-ray tube it is palatal).
(2) Other views—vertex occlusal, lateral cephalogram and PA skull (facial bones).
(3) Adjacent teeth must be examined and tested for vitality.

Exposure

(1) Raise a palatal or labial flap.
(2) Vessels and nerves of the incisive canal can be transected with impunity.
(3) Uncover the crown with burrs or chisel.
(4) If palatal, remove tissue overlying crown and pack with Whitehead's varnish or Coe-Pak. This is removed after 10 days.
(5) If canine is buccally placed and tooth is to be exposed, use an apically repositioned flap.
(6) Where supernumeraries are present, the majority are palatal; remove overlying bone with hand held chisel to prevent damage to adjacent teeth.

Removal and transplantation

The canine may be transplanted if space is available and root form is suitable.

(1) Position the transplanted tooth into the socket created and splint into position for approximately 2 weeks.

(2) Transplanted teeth must be reviewed regularly, watching for root resorption.

Apicectomy and Retrograde Root Filling

This is a surgical aid to endodontics.

Indications

This procedure is indicated for unresolved periapical infection following root canal therapy, periapical cysts, teeth with inaccessible root canals (curved apex, fractured reamers) and over filled root canals.

All teeth requiring apicectomy should, where possible, have orthograde root fillings. Mucoperiosteal flaps may be rectangular, triangular or semilunar, but must be of sufficient size to allow access.

The apical area is curetted and the tooth apicected obliquely in order to enable access to root canal which should be enlarged with a burr and sealed with either amalgam or zinc oxide/eugenol.

Postoperative follow-up radiographs should be taken at 1 week to check the seal. Review at 6 months to check on bone regeneration.

Fraenectomy (Upper Labial)

Indications

This is indicated where a diastema is present between upper centrals and through which the labial fraenum passes and is attached to the incisive papilla.

Method

(1) Pull the upper lip upwards, incise down to bone on either side of the fraenum, which then comes away from the upper lip. This is

removed from the under surface of the upper lip which is then sutured.

(2) The midline suture is cleared of fibrous tissue using a fissure burr or nasal saw.

(3) A Coe-Pak dressing is then placed over the suture for 10 days.

Chapter 8

Orthognathic Surgery

ARRANGEMENTS

(1) Remember that for elective and aesthetic procedures there is no scope for poor planning, errors or omissions.
(2) Look at the admissions list 2 weeks beforehand so that you may confirm any complex operative plan and organise special nursing, physiotherapy, photography or laboratory technical help in theatre or postoperatively.
(3) Check the fixation arrangements and that the splints fit the models.
(4) Notify theatre of any special instruments or other requirements.
(5) For orthodontic fixation, check the availability of brackets, elastics, ligatures and adhesives. Inform orthodontic colleagues of arrangements.

PREOPERATIVE PREPARATION

(1) Take a full general history.
(2) Carry out physical examination.
(3) Investigations—full blood count, urea and electrolytes, blood grouping; save serum or crossmatch whole blood if needed.
(4) Check current radiographs, e.g. lateral cephalogram, panoral and any special views (intraorally of the operative site).
(5) If uncertain of any aspect of a proposed operation, ask your senior clinician. Mention to him early in the working day any snags that you anticipate.
(6) Obtain informed consent—remember that any explanation to the patient must be plain, easily understood and unhurried. Answer the patient's queries honestly, but avoid detailed descriptions of surgical procedures.
(7) Outline principal postoperative events, such as swelling, soreness, jaws wired, difficulty swallowing, minor bleeding. Describe intensive care procedures and mention the feeding problem.
(8) Forewarn the anaesthetist of special airway or other requirements.

(9) Check that the theatre list contains an adequate operative description.
(10) Check the drug sheet, including preoperative night sedation, premedication, antibiotics and steroids.

FITTING SPLINTS

(1) Try in the splints and check that they fit.
(2) Cement the lower splint first.
(3) Dry the teeth and splints scrupulously.
(4) Wax out screw holes and cleats, etc.
(5) Practice your cementing procedure to achieve a thin, even lute of cement.
(6) Mix black copper cement on a cold glass slab; two drops of the liquid per tooth included will be sufficient.
(7) Clean and smooth the splints after cementing (*Note* including the cleats and locking plates).

THEATRE

(1) Arrive early, ensure that sister and the anaesthetist are fully conversant with the operative plan, check the availability of special requirements, reserve fixation equipment, etc.
(2) Display the necessary radiographs, profile plans, and ensure that articulated current models are safely on show.
(3) Finalise arrangements and phone calls well before theatre so that you are not troubled unnecessarily by enquiries and ensure that relevant personnel know where you are (see also Chapter 4).

POSTOPERATIVE
(see also Chapter 4)

(1) Be prepared to accompany the patient to the recovery area and from there to the ward or intensive care area if required.
(2) Issue clear nursing instructions regarding airway or bleeding problems, arrange contact procedure.
(3) Leave wirecutters and clear instructions for the emergency release of fixation.
(4) Ensure that regular aspiration and checks on nasopharyngeal air flow are undertaken.
(5) Arrange regular monitoring of temperature, pulse and blood pressure.

(6) Review the dietary arrangements; ensure adequate fluid input and nutritional requirements, consider intravenous/parenteral/oral methods.
(7) Examine chest and calves daily and organise appropriate physiotherapy.
(8) Check fixation, oral hygiene and prescribe mouthwashes, e.g. bicarbonate in 5 vols hydrogen peroxide for mucolysis.
(9) Review occlusion regularly and remember that the nasopharyngeal airway is a useful suction route, but early removal provides patient comfort.

Investigations

Urea and electrolytes—day 1
Haemoglobin and PCV—day 2 (after equilibration)
Radiographs when ambulant
Manage infective chest or donor site complications by appropriate laboratory investigations (sputum or swab culture and sensitivity) and therapy (? antibiotic change and local treatment).

Follow-Up

Wirecutters (hospital or patient's) and advice on use when discharged.
Suture removal, check occlusion and bone graft site at 7–10 days in out-patient department.
Postoperative OPT, lateral cephalogram (if this is unit policy).
Tape wounds with Steristrips when under tension to avoid scar stretch, e.g. iliac crest.
Ensure discharge summary is sent early to general practitioners.
Encourage patient morale.

OSTEOTOMY SITES

Segmental

(1) Check the operative plan (including any extractions), check splints, locking bars, screws (and screwdrivers) and any templates or occlusal wafers required in theatre. Check the splints (on the models and in the mouth) 1 week preoperatively.

(2) Detailed radiographs of the osteotomy sites must be available. Is occlusal grinding required in theatre?
(3) Circumferential wires—are these needed? Is it planned to use intermaxillary fixation? If so make the necessary recovery arrangements.
(4) Anticipate any problems of segmental movement or anatomy which may complicate induction or maintenance of anaesthesia or the removal of a nasotracheal tube.

Mandibular Ramus

(1) These are generally more significant surgical procedures, made easier with special instruments and retractors, especially when the approach is intraoral. Warn the patient of any possibility of facial nerve weakness or of an external scar, or of lip and tongue paraesthesia, and of the degree of swelling which is likely. Mention any dressings, drain tubes and intravenous infusion sites.
(2) Vertical sub-sigmoid, L and C shaped osteotomies and sagittal split all move the entire dental arch, and the fixation arrangements must therefore allow the repositioned arch to locate firmly onto the upper dental arch directly, or via a wafer (fixation periods and methods vary, whether wires or bolts).
(3) Postoperative radiographs will generally be required to check the position of fragments.
(4) Usual in-patient stay will vary from 3 to 10 days.

Maxillary

(1) In addition to the general items above, warn the patient of expected postoperative swelling and minor nose bleeding and of any possibility of sensory nerve loss in the cheeks or teeth.
(2) Tell them of the likely period of fixation and if a facial frame is likely to be used to fix the mobilised maxillary fragments. Discuss the social difficulties of these, and the danger to nearby people when turning round.

Bimaxillary and Higher Level Midface

(1) If both jaws are to be entirely repositioned, ensure the necessary fixation apparatus is available, e.g. bone-pins, halo, oral projecting bar, universal joints and necessary instruments for their use.

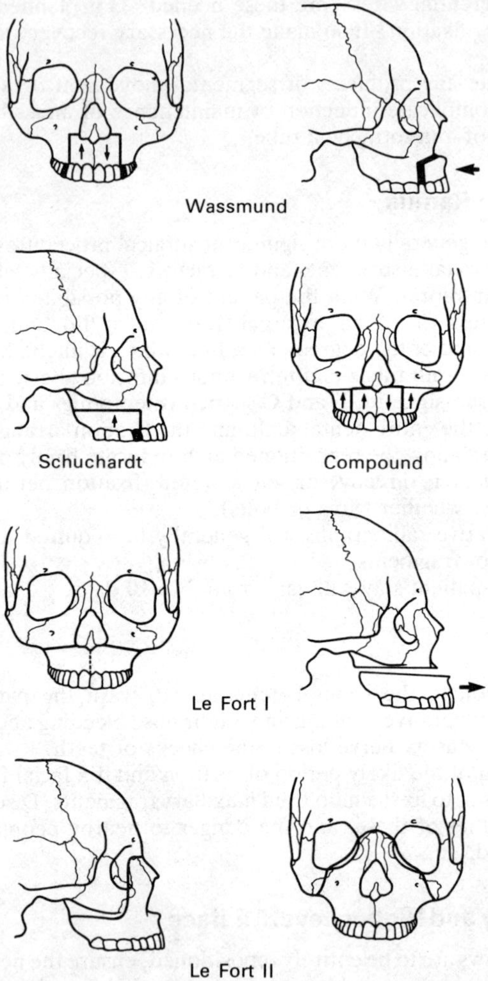

Fig. 8.1 Some maxillary osteotomies.

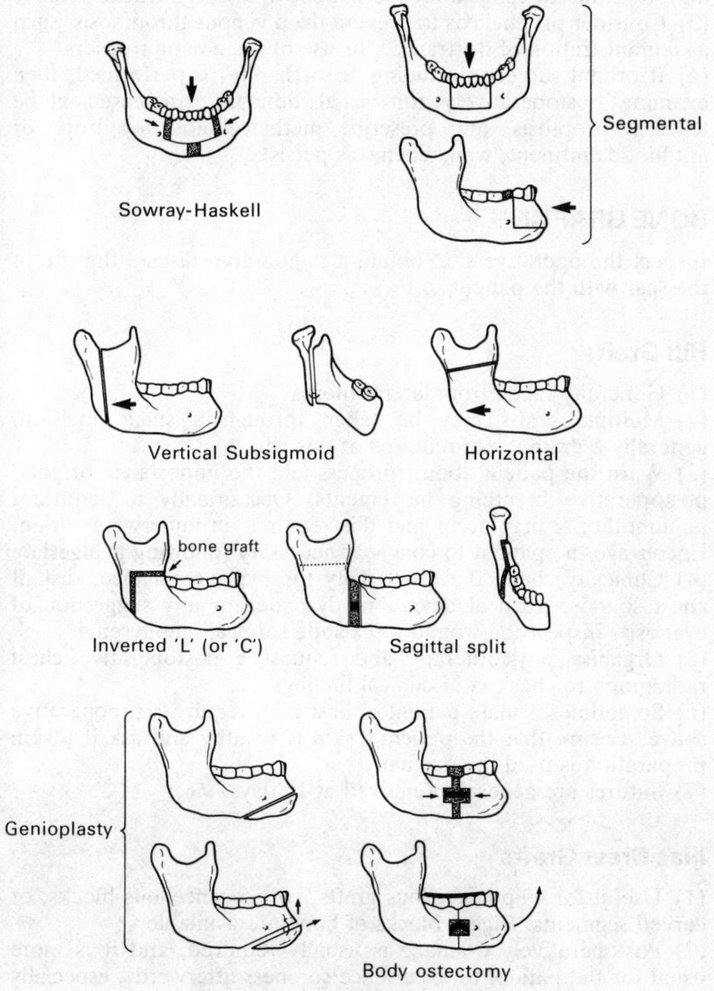

Fig. 8.2 Some mandibular osteotomies.

(2) Additional investigations required are liver function tests, crossmatching more whole blood, e.g. 4 units, chest X-ray, ECG and, if required, consent for the patient to undergo tracheostomy.
(3) Consider prophylaxis to prevent deep venous thrombosis, such as administration of dextran 70, or use of pneumatic trousers.
(4) If orbital surgery (including tarsorrhaphy) is performed, then examine postoperatively for visual difficulty, increased globe tension, proptosis, and prescribe methylcellulose eyedrops or antibiotic ointment, while chemosis persists.

BONE GRAFTING

Inspect the operative site, obtain a radiograph, discuss the site of the scar with the patient.

Rib Grafts

(1) Generally taken from lateral thorax.
(2) Multiple grafts may be taken through a single incision, generally a drain is not required at this site.
(3) Warn the patient about soreness and the importance of good postoperative breathing movements. Occasionally a significant pneumothorax may occur and this requires an underwater drain. Encourage the patient to cough, if necessary following analgesia.
(4) Clinically check the chest daily for hyper-resonance, distant chest sounds, tracheal deviation, dyspnoea or any suggestion of cyanosis. Inspect the wound to exclude surgical emphysema.
(5) Organise physiotherapy and request a postoperative chest radiograph to check your clinical findings.
(6) Sometimes a male patient's chest may require a preoperative shave. Ensure that the patient's skin is healthy and ask if a skin preparation is used in your unit.
(7) Sutures are generally removed at 10 days.

Iliac Crest Grafts

(1) Useful for chip cancellous grafts, corticocancellous blocks, or carved segments. Bigger blocks of bone are available.
(2) Postoperatively drainage is usually required, and it is more usual for the patient to experience soreness afterwards, especially when walking.

(3) X-ray preoperatively if previous graft has been taken from the donor site.
(4) If extensive medial exposure is required at operation, check postoperative bowel sounds, enquire from patient signs of bowel activity (passing wind, borborygmi).
(5) Occasionally patients having a large graft may experience numbness of the lateral cutaneous nerve of the thigh, also urinary retention has been reported occasionally in male patients.
(6) Observe the wound daily for unfavourable signs (swelling, erythema, tenderness or discharge). Ensure a swab is taken if these events should occur.
(7) Mobilise the patient early with appropriate analgesia, arrange any physiotherapy required.
(8) The drain may generally be removed when no longer active (usually after 48 hours). Check that the vacuum is regularly reapplied and the bottle changed as necessary. After drain removal, either leave the wound open or cover it with a light, dry, non-adhesive dressing. Alternatively, ask if it is usual in your unit for a sealant spray to be applied at this stage.
(9) Remember to ask in the out-patient department how the wound is progressing; inspect as required.

Chapter 9

Preprosthetic Surgery

Preprosthetic surgery is carried out to aid the insertion and function of dentures. It involves surgery of the hard and soft tissues and commences with tooth extraction. The edentulous ridge should be stable, retentive and comfortable.

The fitting of immediate dentures involves:
Preparation for alveoloplasty
Mylohyoid ridge reduction
Removal of tori
Soft tissue surgery
Fraeni
Papillary hyperplasia and tuberosity reduction
Vestibuloplasty
Osteotomies
Implants

IMMEDIATE DENTURES

Immediate dentures restore the appearance and allow for immediate function, thus reducing ridge resorption.

General Principles

(1) Perform multiple extractions sequentially, posterior teeth before anterior teeth. Start with mandibular molars, then maxillary molars and finally anterior teeth. Resorption is slower in the mandible.
(2) Perform complicated extractions first, retain alveolar bone and where possible section teeth. Avoid loss of buccal and cortical bone.
(3) Avoid excessive stripping of mucoperiosteum thus minimising resorption.
(4) Excise inflamed interdental papillae.
(5) Avoid decreasing vestibular height by allowing healing by secondary intention rather than primary closure at the expense of sulcus depth.

(6) It is imperative that the operator check that the denture is ready before completing extractions.
(7) After issuing immediate dentures, give instructions regarding their care. They must not be removed for 24 hours after surgery. On removal they must be rinsed and immediately reinserted.

IDEAL EDENTULOUS RIDGE

This is a U-shaped ridge of good height and width, thereby increasing the denture-bearing area. It should be smooth with no sharp edges and should have firm, supportive soft tissue, with elasticity in the peripheral tissues to allow a good seal.

Alveoloplasty

Alveoloplasty is a preparation of the residual ridge for dentures. It can be carried out digitally (compression following extraction) or surgically where irregularities of the ridge are corrected. Buccal and labial alveoloplasty is used to remove undercuts to allow a path for insertion of the denture. In interseptal alveoloplasty the septal bone is removed. Use osteoplastic flaps to preserve and approximate the cortical plates, as this results in less alveolar resorption.

Mylohyoid Ridge Reduction

Sharp, prominent mylohyoid ridges interfere with the lingual flanges of dentures and should be smoothed. A crestal incision avoiding the lingual and mental nerves allows exposure of the ridge. After use of the appropriate flap, the sharp ridge is reduced using an acrylic burr or file.

Excision of Tori

These can occur in the mandible and the maxilla. They slowly increase in size and can interfere with the denture fit and construction. The overlying mucosa is thin and can ulcerate when exposed to pressure from dentures. Ideally, they are removed if large or if the patient is concerned. Take care with palatal tori as oronasal fistulas can be created. The surgeon may request a compression plate.

SOFT TISSUE SURGERY

Fraenectomy

Labial and buccal fraenectomy

(1) Use a diamond excision technique or a Z-plasty.
(2) Maintain the sulcus depth by suturing the mucosa to the underlying periosteum at the depth of the sulcus.
(3) Where a diastema is present, remove the fibrous tissue between the teeth with either a nasal saw or a burr.

Lingual fraenectomy

Lingual fraenectomies can be carried out simply by snipping at the mid-point of the band with scissors or using cutting diathermy.

Maxillary Tuberosity

Enlargements are due to bone or fibrous tissue. Fibrous tissue is usually excised by a wedge resection allowing reduction in vertical and lateral dimensions. If the maxillary ridge is in contact with the mandibular ridge a segmental osteotomy may be necessary to achieve the interarch space. The retromolar pads may also be reduced in size.

Tuberoplasty

Tuberoplasty is effected when the pterygoid hamulus is infractured and the post-tuberosity sulcus is extended by gutta percha lining in the denture.

Inflammatory Hyperplasia

Poor fitting dentures can give rise to flabby ridges. Remove the dentures and adjust them and line the fitting surface with tissue conditioner. The problem may then resolve, but if not excise the base of the hyperplastic lesion with scalpel, scissors or cutting diathermy and allow healing to take place by secondary intention under the soft-lined temporary denture. New dentures are constructed when the tissue has healed.

Papillary Hyperplasia of the Palate

This is caused by poor fitting dentures that are worn continually for 24 hours a day and poor oral hygiene.

Treatment

(1) Improve the oral hygiene, prescribe an antifungal agent, e.g. amphotericin or nystatin.
(2) Use a soft reline material for the denture base.
(3) Surgery is the last resort.
(4) If surgery is carried out remove the tissues supraperiosteally with diathermy or an acrylic burr and allow healing by granulation as for inflammatory hyperplasia.

ALVEOLAR ATROPHY (FLAT RIDGES)

Vestibuloplasty

Vestibuloplasty is carried out when more than 2 cm of bone is present in the midbody of the mandible, the aim being to increase the sulcus depth. In the mandible this can be achieved both buccally and lingually, whereas in the maxilla this can only be carried out buccally.

Methods

(1) *Submucous dissection*—This fixes the oral mucosa in the new deepened sulcus by wiring the dentures in position.
(2) *Supraperiosteal flap*—This allows for repositioning of the sulcus at a new depth. The raw area of connective tissue is allowed to epithelialise.
(3) *Supraperiosteal resection with split skin graft*—The exposed raw area may be covered with a free graft of skin or mucous membrane to facilitate epithelialisation.

Augmentation of Bone Base

Where resorption is extreme and the mandibular body is less than 2 cm in height, the height can be increased by a *visor osteotomy*. The mandible is split in a sagittal direction and the lingual fragment is raised, pedicled on the lingual soft tissue. The vertical height is increased with retention of the alveolar crest. Immediate or delayed vestibuloplasty is required. Interpositional autograft or allograft can be used to improve ridge form.

Skeletal Base Osteotomy

Maxillary and mandibular osteotomies may be carried out prior to the extraction of teeth (and in the edentulous) to minimise denture instability problems, e.g. sagittal split osteotomies for prognathism and retrognathism along with maxillary osteotomies.

Implants

(1) *Subperiosteal*—This is where the framework is placed in a subperiosteal position.
(2) *Mandibular staple bone plate*—An implant is placed intraorally via an extraoral approach and is fixed to the mandible. An overdenture fixes to the intraoral projections.
(3) *Osseointegrated implants*—These implants are tapped and screwed into the maxilla and the mandible. Six months is allowed for osteosynthesis before fitting the superstructure with fixed bridge work.
(4) *Hydroxyapatite*—This is injected subperiosteally and used to eliminate undercuts and increase ridge height.

Chapter 10

Benign Cysts and Odontogenic Tumours

Benign Cysts

ODONTOGENIC EPITHELIUM

Keratocyst (Primordial Cyst)

Keratocysts arise from the dental lamina. The lining is very thin, keratinised epithelium; the capsule often has daughter cysts. They frequently occur in the ramus of the mandible but can be found anywhere. The cysts often reach a large size and can displace teeth. X-ray appearance may show multilocular cysts which resemble an ameloblastoma.

Contents

Dirty white inspissated keratin.
Aspirate contains less than 4 g/100 ml of protein.

Treatment

(1) Depends on size and position.
(2) The cysts can be enucleated, resected with bone grafting or marsupialised.
(3) They are difficult to remove because of the thin lining and capsule containing daughter cysts.
(4) The mucosa over the cyst has a potential for recurrent cyst formation.

Dentigerous Cyst (Follicular Cyst)

Dentigerous cysts are associated with an unerupted tooth crown and are attached at the cementoenamel junction, cystic change occurring in remnants of enamel organ originating from the reduced enamel epithelium. Most frequently found in mandible, they can displace teeth and cause tooth resorption.

Contents

Cholesterol crystals.

Lining

Stratified squamous epithelium.

Treatment

(1) Depends on site, size and the tooth involved.
(2) Enucleation or marsupialisation is employed to allow eruption of displaced tooth.

Eruption Cyst

This is a dentigerous cyst above an unerupted tooth.

Treatment

Deroof the cyst.

Radicular Cyst (Apical and Lateral)

From the activated epithelial cell rests of Malassez, cells form a spongy network which condenses with inflammation giving rise to an epithelial layer and an outer connective tissue layer. These are associated with a non-vital tooth. If the area at the apex of the tooth is >1 cm it is more likely to be a cyst than a granuloma.

Contents

Straw coloured fluid containing cholesterol crystals.
Protein content >5 g/100 ml.

Histology

Stratified squamous epithelium which may become keratinised, goblet cells, hyaline bodies of Rushton.

Treatment

Usually involves enucleation ± retrograde apical seal.

Residual Cyst

A radicular cyst left *in situ* after extraction of a tooth.

Treatment

Enucleation is the usual treatment. Occasionally, marsupialisation aids denture retention.

NON-ODONTOGENIC EPITHELIUM

Nasopalatine Cyst

Nasopalatine cysts arise from epithelium of the nasopalatine duct. Adjacent teeth are vital. The cyst is >7 mm in diameter (normal incisal fossa <7 mm). The median palatine cyst is believed to be a posterior extension of the nasopalatine cyst.

Histology

Stratified squamous epithelium with respiratory epithelium at the nasal end.

Treatment

Enucleation/marsupialisation.

Globulomaxillary Cyst

This is a pear-shaped radiolucency lying between, and occasionally displacing, the roots of the upper lateral incisor and canine. Its origin is obscure.

Treatment

Enucleation.

Median Mandibular Cyst

The existence of this cyst is questionable.

Nasolabial Cyst

Rare, presents as a swelling in soft tissues of the upper lip, 'bracket sign' on radiograph. Its origin is obscure, ? nasolacrimal duct, ? fusion of maxillary and lateral nasal processes.

Treatment

Excision.

CYSTS OF THE SOFT TISSUES

Retention Cyst

Retention cysts have an epithelial lining of ductal origin. It is impossible to distinguish clinically between an extravasation and a retention cyst.

Extravasation Cyst

Extravastion cysts have a connective tissue lining.

Treatment

Retention cysts and extravasation cysts may be treated by:
- Surgical excision
- Cryotherapy
- Electrocoagulation.

Mucocele

This is a retention or extravasation cyst from the minor salivary glands. It is relatively common, often associated with minor trauma.

Ranula

This is a mucocele in the floor of the mouth. It arises from the sublingual gland and occasionally may plunge deep to mylohyoid in an hourglass fashion.

Treatment

Surgical removal of cyst with feeder sublingual gland, or marsupialisation.

Dermoid Cyst

A dermoid cyst often occurs in the floor of mouth, and is lined by stratified squamous epithelium with skin appendages, e.g. hair follicles and sebaceous glands in the fibrous wall. The cyst originates above mylohoid muscle, but may penetrate it. It is often filled with keratin.

Histologically there are three types:

(1) *Epidermoid*—Lined by stratified squamous epithelium and contains keratin.

(2) *Dermoid*—Contains skin appendages, sebaceous glands and hair follicles.

(3) *Teratoid*—Contains ectodermal, endodermal and mesodermal elements.

Treatment

Surgical removal.

NON-EPITHELIAL CYSTS

Solitary Bone Cysts (Simple Bone Cysts, Traumatic Bone Cysts)

A single cyst with no epithelial lining, occurring above the inferior dental canal. The majority are found in the mandible between the canine and third molar region and are asymptomatic. Teeth are vital, characteristically the cyst presents interdentally. The origin may be traumatic.

Contents

Air or serosanguinous fluid.

Treatment

Open cyst and curette/fill with autogenous blood.

Aneurysmal Bone Cyst

This is very rare, pathogenesis probably involving vascular disturbance with features of giant cell granuloma or ossifying/cementifying fibroma. There is a soap bubble appearance on X-ray.

Histology

Blood filled spaces
Multinucleated giant cells
Woven bone

Treatment

Complete curettage or local excision.

Stafne Cavity

This presents as a salivary depression in the body of the mandible, radiolucent appearance; it lies beneath the inferior dental canal.

Treatment

No treatment is required.

EVALUATION

Clinical Examination

Check for:
- Missing teeth
- Displaced teeth
- Root resorption
- Expansion of bone
- Tooth vitality (early cementoma formation may mimic periapical infection)
- Discharging sinuses
- Bluish mucosal swelling
- Anaesthesia or paraesthesia

Radiology

Radiological views include the following:
(1) *Intraoral*—Periapical, standard occlusal, oblique occlusal views.
(2) *Extraoral*—OPG, PA, lateral, lateral oblique, 15° + 45° occipitomental views, ± tomography.
The cysts appear as radiolucent areas with a thin radio-opaque

compact bone surround. Remember that tumorous lesions can simulate cysts.

Aspiration

(1) Anaesthetise the area; aspirate using a strong wide-bore needle.
(2) There is a risk of infection postaspiration; so one must be ready to operate if necessary.
(3) Radicular and dentigerous cysts contain a straw-coloured fluid sparkling with cholesterol.
(4) Aspirate may be submitted for electrophoresis.
Keratocysts contain <4 g/100 ml of soluble protein, radicular and dentigerous cysts contain >5 g/100 ml of soluble protein. If blood is aspirated suspect presence of aneurysmal bone cyst or central cavernous haemangioma. If air is aspirated suspect maxillary sinus, or traumatic bone cyst.

Treatment of Cysts

Untreated cysts can increase in size leading to fracture or damage to adjoining structures. Cystic specimens should be examined histologically.

Types of treatment

Enucleation
Marsupialisation

Enucleation

This is a one step procedure; wide exposure is required with the flap based on solid bone, careful dissection of the complete lining is needed. The pathological specimen must be complete. The flap is then replaced or packed into bone cavity and the specimen sent for pathological examination.

Marsupialisation

This is employed where the cyst is large and there is minimal bone support. This process preserves vitality of adjacent teeth and allows normal eruption of teeth also avoiding damage to the inferior dental nerve. The cyst may be excised later. In mixed dentition, marsupialisation is preferred to enucleation because of the preservation of dentition. The cyst lining becomes confluent with oral mucous membrane and may become normal stratified squamous epithelium. The *disadvantages* include the fact that the specimen is not complete, and that this treatment requires prolonged follow-up.

Helpful Surgical Tips

(1) Plan surgery.
(2) Adequately expose cyst.
(3) Design flap edges to rest eventually on solid bone.
(4) Minimise bleeding to prevent breakdown of flap.
(5) Avoid tearing of cyst lining, this can prevent recurrence.
(6) Strip cyst with gauze swab, using non-toothed dissecting forceps to prevent damage to the histological specimen.
(7) Where the inferior dental nerve is exposed, avoid neurolytic agents, e.g. Whitehead's varnish, and minimise trauma to avoid prolonged paraesthesia.
(8) Where a large cyst leads to possibility of fractured jaw, preoperative splints may be needed.

Odontogenic Tumours

Odontogenic tumours are hamartomas or neoplasms arising from the dental lamina or its derivatives. Generally they are slow growing, occur within the jaws and are benign. There are three groups of odontogenic tumours.

(1) *Epithelial*
Ameloblastoma
Adenomatoid odontogenic tumour
Calcifying epithelial odontogenic tumour (Pindborg tumour)

(2) *Mesenchymal*
Cementoma—Gigantiform cementoma, periapical cemental dysplasia, cementifying fibroma, benign cementoblastoma

(3) *Mixed epithelial and odontogenic tumours*
Ameloblastic fibroma (fibroameloblastoma)
Odontomes

EPITHELIAL

Ameloblastoma (Various Types)

This is the most aggressive of the odontogenic tumours; it is slowly invasive but does not metastasise; it originates from the dental lamina or its derivatives. Of these tumours 80% are mandibular and 20% are maxillary, the majority occurring in the molar area. They are slow growing, multilocular or unilocular radiolucencies on X-ray, and the bony septa give a soap bubble appearance.

Microscopically, the tumours appear as islands or sheets of ameloblast-like cells with central stellate reticulum-like cells.

Treatment

Surgical resection.

Adenomatoid Odontogenic Tumour (Adenoameloblastoma)

This occurs in the second decade of life, with a female predominance; there is premaxillary involvement. These tumours are often associated with impacted teeth hence they are often mistaken for follicular cysts. These tumours may be encapsulated.

Microscopically, they are duct-like structures lined by columnar cells.

Treatment

Conservative curettage is the only treatment. These tumours do not recur.

Calcifying Epithelial Odontogenic Tumour (Pindborg Tumour)

The site of origin is reduced enamel epithelium from an unerupted tooth.

Microscopically, they are polyhedral epithelial cells with eosinophilic globules which calcify. They are mainly mandibular, radiolucent lesions with spicules of calcification.

Treatment

Excision with a margin of healthy tissue.

MESENCHYMAL

Cementoma

These are lesions in which the predominant feature is the presence of tissue which looks like cementum. Tumours cover a wide spectrum. There are four distinct entities.

Gigantiform cementoma
Periapical cemental dysplasia
Cementifying fibroma
Benign cementoblastoma (true cementoma)

Gigantiform cementoma

This is rare, most common in negro women, and present as irregular radio-opaque masses which are bilateral with symmetrical distribution. They are not fused to adjacent bone.

If asymptomatic leave alone, but progressive growth can cause jaw expansion and deformity.

Periapical cemental dysplasia

Tends to involve periapical tissues of many teeth, but can affect only lower incisors. It appears in the periapical area and has a life-cycle commencing with radiolucency going through to radio-opacity.

No treatment is required.

Cementifying fibroma

This is a benign neoplasm which may be encapsulated.

Microscopically, it is made up of cellular fibroblastic tissue with calcified masses. It is not related to teeth apices and is similar to ossifying fibroma, both being identical clinically and radiographically.

Treatment involves conservative excision.

Benign cementoblastoma (true cementoma)

This occurs usually in young people, and is more common in the mandible. It is associated with the roots of one tooth usually premolar or molar, and has a radio-opaque appearance. The mass is attached to the tooth root; resorption is often seen. The tendency to expand should thus be removed.

Odontogenic Myxoma

This is a destructive neoplasm arising from the jaw bone, usually in young people. It is indistinguishable radiologically from ameloblastoma as it shows multilocular radiolucency. Differential diagnosis includes ameloblastoma, odontogenic cysts or giant cell lesions.

At operation the tissue is soft, pale and mucinous. Although benign, it is difficult to eliminate hence the recurrence rate of 80%.

Microscopically, it shows fibroblasts in mucoid ground substance.

Treatment

This involves wide excision.

Odontogenic Fibroma

This is a slow growing encapsulated tumour of fibroblasts that occurs in the second decade of life with a greater incidence in the mandible rather than the maxilla. It is asymptomatic and always associated with impacted teeth, hence it resembles a dentigerous cyst.

Microscopically, there are streaks of epithelial cells with areas of calcification, resembling cementum or dysplastic bone.

Treatment

Enucleation.

MIXED EPITHELIAL AND ODONTOGENIC TUMOURS

Ameloblastic Fibroma

A true mixed tumour in which epithelial and mesenchymal elements are neoplastic. Less common than the ameloblastoma, however it clinically and radiologically resembles the ameloblastoma. Found in the younger age group this tumour is locally invasive and aggressive but does not metastasise.

Treatment

Local excision, rarely resection.

Odontomes (Compound, Complex)

Composed of hard dental tissues, these may occur at any age and are slow growing. There are two types on radiological examination:
(1) *Compound*—multiple denticles.
(2) *Complex*—disorganised irregular mass of dentine, enamel and cementum. There is no recognisable tooth form.
Both types can prevent tooth eruption.

Treatment

Removal of tumour.

Chapter 11

Oral Malignancy

Malignancy within the oral cavity accounts for approximately 2400 new cases each year in the United Kingdom and comprises about 1–2% of all cancer. It is more common from the fifth and sixth decades onwards, but does present in young people. It is remarkably evenly distributed and comprises predominantly squamous cell carcinomas. Despite the general public's awareness of cancer, and the ready accessibility of the mouth to examination, oral cancer is still seen presenting late. Thus, the prognosis has not greatly improved over the last two decades. The underlying aetiology of oral malignancy is, as yet, unclear whereas certain conditions are known to have a premalignant potential. The role of the houseman in the management of malignant disease is chiefly concerned with the recognition of the disease (which may be totally unsuspected) and the management of the patient preoperatively and postoperatively.

Table 11.1
Oral Lesions with Malignant Potential

Type	*Percentage undergoing malignant change*
Erythroplakia	?80
Leukoplakia	
Homogeneous	0–0.5
Verrucous	4–6
Erosive	? 10
Speckled	20–30
Sublingual keratosis	50

PRINCIPAL PREDISPOSING CONDITIONS FOR PRECANCER

Iron deficiency
Vitamin B deficiency

Oral submucous fibrosis
Lichen planus (erosive form)
Syphilis etc.

CONDITIONS WITH ASSOCIATED ORAL SIGNS HAVING MALIGNANT POTENTIAL ELSEWHERE

Gardner's syndrome
Peutz–Jegher's syndrome
Gorlin's syndrome

CLASSIFICATION OF MALIGNANCIES AFFECTING THE ORAL CAVITY

Primary Carcinomas

(1) Primary carcinoma of a surface—mainly squamous cell carcinoma, rarely malignant melanoma.
(2) Primary carcinoma of a gland—usually salivary gland, including the widely distributed minor glands.
(3) Intrabony tumours arising from epithelial remnants, e.g. a cyst.

Secondary Carcinomas

(1) Secondary carcinoma within lymph nodes—e.g. a cervical node metastasis from a tumour of the tongue.
(2) Secondary carcinoma within bone—e.g. carcinomas of breast with secondary deposit in mandible.
(3) Secondary carcinoma on the mucosa—e.g. surface deposit of malignant carcinoma of the bronchus.

Primary Sarcoma

(1) Primary sarcoma in bone—e.g. osteosarcoma or chondrosarcoma
(2) Primary sarcoma in muscle—e.g. rhabdomyosarcoma

Reticuloses

(1) Lymphatic (2) Leukaemic deposits }	May be found in the hard and soft tissues around the jaws

It can be appreciated that malignancy affecting the mouth may arise from oral mucosa or the bone of the jaws, or it may intrude from surrounding structures, such as the maxillary antrum, nose or salivary glands. It may also be part of a generalised process of secondary spread. The clinical implications of these facts must be borne in mind and the importance of a general examination can be clearly appreciated.

CLINICAL EXAMINATION AND HISTORY

Malignant change within the mouth has a variable presentation. It is usually symptomless. As a general rule, if doubt persists as to a clinical diagnosis, it is wiser to biopsy suspicious areas of mucosa. Clinically, intraoral carcinomas may present as persistent ulceration, leukoplakia, erythroplakia or exophytic growths.

(1) Dentures should always be removed before starting the examination. Two mirrors often help in retracting the lips, cheeks and tongue. The lips should be examined with the mouth open and closed. Any alteration in colour, texture or surface abnormalities should be noted and then digital palpation carried out.

(2) The labial commissures and buccal mucosa are best examined with the mouth wide open, using the mirrors as retractors. The dorsum of the tongue is best inspected with the mouth partially open. The patient should then protrude the tongue and its mobility should be noted. With the aid of mirrors, retract the tongue and inspect its lateral surfaces. The ventral surface is best viewed with the tip of the tongue touching the vault of the palate. It is of considerable help to hold the tip of the tongue with gauze in order to adequately examine its posterior and posterolateral aspects, and for biopsy purposes.

(3) Examine the floor of the mouth, while the tongue is still elevated, especially the lingual pouch area. The hard and soft palates together with the retromandibular region including the tonsillar fossa can be inspected with the mouth wide open, the patient's head tilted backwards and the tongue gently depressed with a wooden spatula.

(4) Bimanual palpation of the submandibular and submental triangles is an essential part of the oral examination. This is followed by a careful examination of the lymphatic drainage on both sides of the neck.

(5) Stand behind the patient, whose neck should be slightly flexed and whose clothes should be loosened until the points of the shoulders are accessible. Begin palpation with the index fingers on both

mastoid processes and work down the trapezius muscles until they meet the clavicle. Palpate the posterior triangles. Then palpate along the sternomastoid muscle, gripping the muscle between the thumb (posteriorly) and index finger (anteriorly) to check for lymph nodes which lie beneath the muscle and are about 1.25 cm deep to the skin surface. Continue your examination anteriorly to finally include a thorough palpation of the submandibular and submental triangles.

DIFFERENTIAL DIAGNOSIS OF NECK SWELLINGS

Take a careful history prior to a systematic examination, noting the patient's age, whether pain is present and the duration, the site, number and consistency of the neck lumps. If the lump is thought to be a lymph node, check the anatomical area drained by the node in question.

Table 11.2
Useful Investigations of Neck Lumps

Method	*Test*
Haematology	Haemoglobin estimation Full blood count
Radiology	Radiographs of the teeth, jaws, sinuses, chest [Ultrasound investigation]
Bacteriology and virology	Bacterial culture of swabs Tests for infectious mononucleosis, toxoplasmosis, syphilis, tuberculosis Culture biopsy for tuberculosis
Histopathology	Fine needle aspiration cytology Definitive biopsy

SOME HISTOLOGICAL FEATURES OF ORAL CANCER AND PREMALIGNANT LESIONS

Epithelial Dysplasia

This includes loss of polarity of basal cells, increased nuclear/cytoplasmic ratio, increased number of mitotic figures and reduction of cellular cohesion.

Table 11.3
A Classification of Neck Lumps

<table>
<tr><td rowspan="4">Lymph nodes</td><td rowspan="2">Infective</td><td>Bacterial</td><td>Consider tuberculosis, syphilis, head and neck infections etc.</td></tr>
<tr><td>Viral</td><td>Consider infectious mononucleosis, rubella etc.</td></tr>
<tr><td rowspan="2">Malignant</td><td>Primary node pathology</td><td>Lymphomas</td></tr>
<tr><td>Secondary pathology</td><td>Secondary deposits in nodes</td></tr>
<tr><td>Cystic swellings</td><td colspan="3">Dermoids, thyroglossal cyst, branchial cyst, cystic hygroma, sebaceous cyst</td></tr>
<tr><td>Miscellaneous</td><td colspan="3">Carotid body tumour, thyroid enlargements, cervical rib, sternomastoid tumour</td></tr>
</table>

Carcinoma *in situ*

A lesion in which the whole thickness of the epithelium shows malignant cellular features including loss of polarity and stratification, hyperchromatic nuclei which may show variations in size and shape, increased nuclear/cytoplasmic ratio and nucleoli which are enlarged and often multiple. Mitoses usually occur in all parts of the epithelium, but invasion is absent.

Squamous Cell Carcinoma

Irregular nests, columns or strands of malignant epithelial cells, infiltrating subepithelially. The tumour cells may resemble any or all of the layers of stratified squamous epithelium. There are frequent variations which may be described histologically, e.g. spindle cell carcinoma when the cells are so shaped but may still show foci of keratinisation.

Verrucous Carcinoma

The appearance and clinical behaviour is distinctive. It shows a low degree of malignancy and is markedly exophytic, eroding rather than invading underlying tissues, including bone. Histologically it is characterised by large, heavily keratinised fronds with bulbous rete pegs which occasionally show degeneration. Mitoses are infrequent.

TNM STAGING OF ORAL CANCER

This shorthand system helps in the planning of treatment and assessment of prognosis:

- **T**—Extent of primary tumour
- **N**—Condition of regional lymph nodes
- **M**—Presence or absence of distant metastases

This classification applies to the anterior two-thirds of the tongue, floor of mouth, buccal mucosa, the alveolar processes and hard palate.

T—Primary tumour

- **TIS**—Carcinoma *in situ*
- **T0**—No evidence of primary tumour
- **T1**—Tumour <2 cm
- **T2**—>2 cm and <4 cm
- **T3**—>4 cm

N—Regional lymph nodes

- **N0**—Regional nodes not palpable
- **N1**—Movable unilateral nodes
  - **N1a**—Nodes considered not to contain tumour
  - **N1b**—Nodes considered to contain tumour
- **N2**—Movable contralateral or bilateral nodes
  - **N2a**—Nodes considered not to contain tumour
  - **N2b**—Nodes considered to contain tumour
- **N3**—Fixed nodes

M—Distant metastases

- **M0**—No evidence of metastases
- **M1**—Distant metastases present

Based on the above variables, the tumour may be staged from stages 1 to 4.

A PREOPERATIVE SCHEDULE

(1) *History*—General medical health, current medication and history of past operations; specific history of the tumour.

(2) *Examination*—General examination, local examination, TNM classification; evidence of spread.

(3) *Radiology*—Specific X-rays may be indicated. Assess evidence for bony invasion. Take an orthopantomogram if facilities are available, alternatively lateral oblique films and intraoral views are usually sufficient for the examination of the mandible. The maxilla, maxillary antrum and nose may be viewed with an orthopantomogram, 15° and 45° occipitomental and lateral skull films. Intraoral films should also be obtained. Tomography and CT scanning may be required to assess the spread of the tumour, particularly when the ethmoid region or the pterygomaxillary space are involved. A chest radiograph is required to act as a baseline during postoperative management and to exclude a possible further primary or secondary tumour.

(4) *Laboratory investigations*

Full blood count and haemoglobin estimation

Test electrolytes, and creatinine in certain cases, particularly when chemotherapy is involved

Liver function tests

Urine analysis

Sickle cell testing if appropriate

(5) *Blood transfusion*—It is wise to crossmatch 3–4 units if extensive surgery is planned, but in all instances the patient's blood should be taken for grouping and the serum saved in case an unexpected transfusion becomes necessary.

(6) *Bacteriology*—Take a sample of sputum and throat swab ± urine analysis as indicated. Evidence of infection is shown by microscopy and culture of swabs—may require specific antibiotic therapy.

(7) *Electrocardiogram*—Usually required since the patients are frequently elderly and should, therefore, be admitted sufficiently early to allow adequate preoperative assessment.

(8) *Teeth*—The condition of the teeth and periodontal tissues must be assessed very carefully to plan the care of the dentition in relation to the treatment plan, remembering the problems which may be associated with radiation caries following extensive radiotherapy to the mouth. Where extensive surgery is to be carried out, the retention of all sound teeth may be mandatory to aid prosthetic rehabilitation. Conversely, if extensive radiotherapy is given to either jaw, careful consideration must be given to extracting teeth within the radiation field. This is particularly

pertinent to teeth in the mandible, since only exceptionally should teeth be retained which are in the field of radiation.

(9) *Anaesthetist*—Telephone the anaesthetist the day before operation, when you have the investigation results in front of you, in order to discuss the case with him.

(10) *Intensive care unit*—This should be booked in advance, if required. After surgery has been carried out, particular care is required in the immediate and early postoperative period.

POSTOPERATIVE CARE

(1) *Postoperative observations*—Pulse, respiratory rate, and blood pressure should be recorded half-hourly for the first 24 hours. The patient's temperature should be recorded 4-hourly and continuous ECG monitoring may be appropriate in certain cases. The house surgeon should be informed of any abnormalities noted in these measurements and appropriate treatment carried out. Examine the patient regularly for possible bleeding under the flaps, as this may jeopardise the surgery if passed unnoticed. Where patients have a bilateral neck dissection, watch for a falling pulse rate and rising blood pressure, as this may indicate cerebral oedema. This must be treated urgently with steroids or with a rapid intravenous infusion of 200 ml of 25% mannitol.

(2) *Fluid balance*—Input and output charts must be kept from the earliest time possible postoperatively. Input is often through an intravenous drip ± a nasogastric tube. Electrolyte measurements may be required regularly.

(3) *Drains*—Usually of a suction type, are absolutely critical to prevent haematomas which may lead to flap breakdown. Drains are removed when the drainage has stopped.

(4) *Medication*

(i) *Antibiotics*—May be required if the pharynx or mouth have been opened, to prevent the possible ingress of commensal organisms. Treat established infection, after the results of a swab.

(ii) *Analgesia*—Regular, frequent low doses are more effective than large doses on demand (prn).

(iii) *Antiemetics*—As required.

(iv) *Sedation*—As indicated.

(5) *Removal of sutures*—Depends on the site and type of suture material. Discuss timing with your registrar or consultant.

(6) *Mobilisation*—generally within 72 hours and usually the earlier the better.

Tracheostomy

Knowledge of specific after-care is essential.
(1) *Immediate after-care*—A trained nurse is required to be in attendance for 24–48 hours. The patient may be humidified and sterile suction must be regularly carried out.
(2) *Fixation of the tube*—The tube should be secured with tapes around the neck or skin sutures. If not secured in place, there is a real danger it may be coughed out.
(3) *Changing the tube*—This must be carried out regularly to prevent the accumulation of mucus within the lumen. Learn how to change the tube on the ward under the supervision of your senior registrar.

Long-term Postoperative Problems to Be Kept Under Review

(1) Loss of self-confidence, depression and rejection by family and friends, following treatment.
(2) Xerostomia, following radiation—Explain importance of excellent oral hygiene and saliva substitutes.
(3) Prosthetic rehabilitation—May require sophisticated obturators etc.
(4) Speech difficulties
(5) Recurrent disease—Maintain clinical vigilance through regular out-patient appointments, e.g. monthly for the first year, bimonthly for the second year, etc.
(6) Trismus
(7) Drooling

Chapter 12

Facial Pain

The case history is the most important single step in diagnosis. After a complete history has been obtained, you should be well on the way to establishing a differential diagnosis and thus a guide to examination and special tests required.

The history should include:

(1) Location of pain—Ask the patient to point to painful area.
(2) Duration—Minutes → years.
(3) Type—Described as sharp, dull, throbbing etc.
(4) Onset—Insidious or specific.
(5) Severity—Best judged by asking if it interferes with everyday activities or sleep. What relief is obtained by analgesics?
(6) Exacerbations and remissions—Does the pain come and go? Are there any initiating factors? Is it worse in the morning or after eating?
(7) Radiation—Record where the pain radiates to.
(8) Associated pathology—Note history of previous pathology in the area under question. Any previous operations at this site?

FACTORS INFLUENCING THE PATIENT'S REACTION TO PAIN

(1) The patient's individual pain threshold
(2) Anxiety states and depression
(3) Fear of ? underlying cause
(4) Duration of pain and loss of sleep
(5) Other chronic illness

SOURCES OF OROFACIAL PAIN

(1) Teeth and supporting structures—Pulpal, periodontal and bone pain. Mucosal lesions, e.g. aphthous ulcers, pemphigus and geographical tongue. Denture trauma.
(2) Neighbouring structures
Temporomandibular joint—Pain dysfunction, arthritic
Paranasal sinuses—Infection and neoplasia

Nose—Middle turbinate septum syndrome
Throat—Eagle syndrome, ossified styloid
Ears—Otitis externa or media
Salivary glands—Infection, duct stricture, calculi
Tonsils—Infection

(3) Referred pain, e.g.
Angina pectoris
Cervical spondylitis

(4) The neuralgias
Primary, e.g. trigeminal, glossopharyngeal
Secondary—Extracranial, e.g. pituitary tumours and carotid aneurysms

(5) Vascular pains, e.g.
Migraine
Cluster headache
Giant cell arteritis

(6) Muscular pains, e.g.
Masseteric hypertrophy
Tension headache

(7) Pain frequently associated with a psychogenic component
Atypical facial pain
Oral dysaesthesia—Glossodynia, xerostomia, persistent bad taste (with no cause found)
Bruxism

INVESTIGATIONS

These will entirely depend on the findings in both the history and examination. They should be carried out systematically until the diagnosis is established. Patients may require referral to other specialists to exclude pain arising in fields outside your department's expertise.

TREATMENT—DEPENDENT ON THE ESTABLISHED DIAGNOSIS

It is well to remember that there is a group of patients who do not respond to simple treatments and persist with chronic facial pain, of uncertain aetiology. Some of these patients have pain of differing origins with a marked psychological component. They are best dealt with by the most senior clinicians!

Chapter 13

Temporomandibular Joint Disorders

The temporomandibular joints function, uniquely in the body, as paired joints throughout the lifetime of an individual. The anatomy is described in detail in most standard texts. In essence it is a diarthrodial joint with upper and lower joint spaces divided by a disc of fibrocartilage. The anterior and posterior thickened bands of the disc and the arrangement of the laminated fibres in the vascular retrodiscal zone have assumed fresh significance in the understanding of clicking and locking in the joint, with an increase in knowledge of the role of the disc in pain and dysfunction syndromes involving these joints. As understanding of the function and pathology of the joint has increased, so has the effectiveness of management of many of the clinical problems.

While the temporomandibular joints are susceptible to the whole range of disorders which affect other joints of the body, the effects of pain or limitation on opening of the mouth often produce more anxiety in patients who are concerned about their ability to speak, chew and breathe with ease and comfort. Evaluation of the patient with temporomandibular disorders, therefore, requires an approach that directs itself to the total patient; joint symptoms may be but one manifestation of a systemic disorder that requires more extensive therapy than the local treatment of one affected joint.

The diagnostic protocol for evaluation of the patient with temporomandibular problems may include: detailed history, physical examination (general and local) and study of the dental occlusion.

EXAMINATION OF THE JOINT

(1) Study opening movement and total range of motion, centrally and laterally.
(2) Observe any deviation in pathway of opening or closing.
(3) Observe joint sounds such as clicking or grating.
(4) Palpate for sensitivity over joint and in external auditory meatus with joint moving and at rest.

EXAMINATION OF MUSCLES

(1) Palpate all relevant muscles of mastication by external and intraoral approaches.
(2) Feel for pain or spasm in the lateral pterygoid by gentle palpation with the little finger behind the maxillary tuberosity.

EXAMINATION OF OCCLUSION

(1) Observe, directly, all obvious occlusal interference.
(2) Use adhesive occlusal wax over lower teeth to check for interceptive contacts in centric or grinding occlusion.
(3) Mark contacts with crayon applied through perforated area in occlusal wax and identify position precisely on dental chart.
(4) Occlusal analysis with mounted casts is occasionally desirable.

RADIOGRAPHIC EXAMINATION

(1) Panoramic radiography, in mouth closed and open positions (conventional and 'high' OPG) usually sufficient for screening and routine diagnosis.
(2) Reverse OPG may provide more information on condyle/fossa relationships.
(3) Transpharyngeal, transcranial oblique and transorbital views are occasionally needed.
(4) Reverse Towne's view provides the best anteroposterior projection of condylar head and neck, especially if fractured.
(5) Tomography, arthrography with contrast medium (e.g. Hypaque), CT scan and scintigraphy are reserved for examination of complex cases.

Radiographic examination provides information on the range of movement in the joint, the position, shape and quality of the bone of the condylar head, the dimension of the overall joint space and a comparison of one side with the other; and, occasionally, osteophytes or foreign bodies within the joint space. Radiographic assessment of the disc is difficult; arthrography, especially double contrast arthrography (medium plus air) is the best method yet available. Blink-mode CT scan and new generation NMR may prove to be as valuable without provoking pain and stiffness.

The most useful function of temporomandibular joint (TMJ) radiography is to interpret the effects of trauma on the joint. The extent of ankylosis is well demonstrated by tomography and CT scan, as is the rare benign or neoplastic lesion of the TMJ. As the large majority of cases of TMJ pain and dysfunction involves minimal observable changes in the hard tissues of the joint, the benefits of radiographic examination are seldom great, except for the exclusion of fracture, dislocation, severe degenerative changes, ankylosis or tumours.

For practical purposes, TMJ problems can be separated into acute or chronic management issues.

ACUTE PROBLEMS

Usually present with severe pain and considerable limitation of opening of the jaw (trismus). It should be remembered that not all cases of trismus are caused by disorders of the joint. Infection of such adjacent structures as the periodontium, submasseteric, temporal and peritonsillar spaces, and acute parotitis, may all produce acute trismus and pain referred to the TMJ and ear.

Classification of Acute TMJ Problems

(1) Traumatic injury
- (i) Fracture, fracture dislocations, joint space effusions, capsular and muscular sprains
- (ii) Dislocation
- (iii) Acute myofascial pain dysfunction syndrome

(2) Infection of intra or periarticular tissues (gonococcal, streptococcal)

(3) Systemic disorders—Gout, tetanus

(4) Functional disorders—Hysterical trismus, acute anorexia nervosa

(5) Tumours of TMJ—May provide acute management problems until diagnosed otherwise.

Fractures Involving TMJ

Most fractures involve the condylar neck and are extra-articular. In children, fractures are often 'greenstick', without displacement. Intracapsular fracture of the condylar head may occur at any age but is rare in adults. The complete articular surface may be crushed to fragments, or a section (often medial) may shear off and become displaced. Except when associated with penetrating injuries, condylar fractures are 'closed'. Fractures of the condyle through the neck may be undisplaced, moderately displaced or dislocated by the pull of the pterygoid muscle into the sphenomaxillary fossa. Rarely, the condyle may be impacted, or dislocated into the middle cranial fossa with fracture of the glenoid fossa. Unilateral condylar fractures, without displacement, show few clinical signs of disturbance except local pain and swelling. When displacement is present there is usually a deviation of the jaw to the affected side on opening. Pain, ecchymosis, swelling and external auditory meatus (EAM) bleeding may also be present. The occlusion may be disturbed. Bilateral condylar fractures, with displacement, produce the Guardsman phenomenon of retrusion of the chin with anterior open bite. Remember that blows to the chin are frequently associated with *contre-coup* fractures of the condylar neck. In all cases of traumatic injury to the face and jaws, fracture of the condyles should be suspected.

Deviation of the jaw on opening or retrusion of the chin or alteration of the bite in the absence of other fractures, and inability to palpate the condylar head on examination with the little finger in the EAM makes radiographic examination by OPG (with, perhaps a Towne's view also) mandatory.

Principles of management of condylar fractures

Greenstick and intracapsular fractures should receive a period of rest, or soft diet, for 2–3 days, followed by early active movements. If stiffness increases, graduated efforts should be made to increase the range of motion. Condyle neck fractures with minimal or no displacement should be treated similarly. Occlusal adjustment may be required at intervals to reduce interceptive contacts. When the condyle is displaced or dislocated, intermaxillary fixation may be employed to hold teeth in occlusion for 10–14 days. This must be followed by self-administered heat and mild exercises to encourage full movement.

Bilateral fractures with condyle head dislocation may require longer periods of intermaxillary fixation, or even direct surgical osteosynthesis to restore the vertical dimension of the face and re-establish normal occlusion.

Traumatic injury to the TMJ without evidence of fracture, but associated with pain and trismus, is usually diagnosed as an effusion, a sprain or a strain. These present all the symptoms found in the sprained ankle; treatment is local warmth, rest and perhaps NSAIDs for 3–4 days followed by remedial exercises to encourage normal movement.

Dislocation of the Condyle

May be spontaneous or traumatic, unilateral or bilateral. Habitual dislocation may occur in attention-seekers (in younger age groups) and in elderly institutionalised patients on phenothiazine-type major tranquillisers.

Reduction is speedily achieved by the injection of 1.5 ml local anaesthetic with vasoconstrictor in the posterior superior dental block site. Wait 10 minutes; if the dislocation has not been reduced by spontaneous relaxation of the contracted temporal and pterygoid muscles, apply gentle downward and backward force to the lower molar regions with the forefingers, when the desired reduction is effected.

Excess force in reducing dislocation may tear and weaken capsular ligaments, promoting habitual dislocation. Frequent dislocation may warrant local injection of the suitable sclerosant (STD) periarticularly on affected side(s). Rarely, surgical procedures such as eminectomy, condylotomy or Dautrey's operation may be necessary.

Acute Myofascial Pain Dysfunction Syndrome

This is most common in young adults. Females predominate 4:1. It usually presents with pain and severe restriction of opening which has appeared on awakening; often preceded by clicking of affected joint and chronic pain of variable duration. Referred pain in ear and face is common. There is occasional history of bruxism or clenching, and presenting deep anterior overbite. Lateral pterygoid on affected side exquisitely painful. Adequate history almost invariably confirms diagnosis; radiographic examination seldom contributory; arthrogram or CT scan may show fixed anterior dislocation of intra-articular disc.

Treatment

(1) Explanation of nature of muscle spasm and local and referred pain.
(2) Reassurance of non-sinister nature of condition.

(3) Topical ethylchloride spray or periarticular infiltration of local anaesthetic to relax muscle spasm.
(4) Local warmth, gentle remedial exercises and non-steroidal anti-inflammatory analgesics are all useful.
(5) Regular review of condition to ensure that treatment is effective and that normal movements are returning.
(6) Anxiety may be treated by small doses of minor tranquillisers at bedtime for 7–14 days. Stelazine 1 mg nightly is better than Valium 5 mg.
(7) Once mouth opening has returned, regular remedial exercises and removal of obvious interceptive contacts maintains progress. Recalcitrant cases with chronic symptoms may benefit from intermittent use of an upper bite plane or soft lower occlusal splint.
(8) Review regularly. If symptoms persist in acute form, reconsider diagnosis.

TMJ Infection

Acute pyogenic arthritis in the joint is extremely rare in the absence of osteomyelitis, actinomycosis, or penetrating wound. If suspected, aspirate pus from joint space for microbiological examination.

Systemic-linked Trismus

Gouty subjects may present with acute pain in TMJ; history is usually confirmatory and response to a short period of indomethacin treatment, when not contraindicated, is usually dramatic. Rarely, psoriatic arthritis may produce restricted opening when psoriasis is of long standing. Tetanus, after a penetrating, contaminated wound, may rarely present as increasing trismus, associated with neck stiffness. When the possibility of this diagnosis exists, admit to intensive care for respiratory care, wound debridement, antitoxin, antibiotics.

Psychological Trismus

The relationship between stress, psychological illness and TMJ pain dysfunction is often discussed but seldom clarified. Occasionally patients see this condition as a way of assisting or modifying an unpleasant life situation. Trismus calls attention to their plight, and enables them to avoid responsibilities. Before concluding that hysteria or neurosis is causative, consider whether acute or chronic TMJ pain has led to or contributed to the emotional state perceived on examination. Where psychological factors appear paramount, or where inability to open mouth may be limited to a desire not to eat, as in anorexia nervosa, provide ample time for investigation and counselling. Most TMJ pain dysfunction is multifactorial in origin, with a threshold; removal of one or more noxious factors usually returns the patient to the 'comfortable' side of the pain threshold. When stress and psychogenic factors are predominant, the diagnostic battle is often won or lost in the first skirmish; if time for counselling is short, reappoint to discuss the problem in detail, without haste.

Tumours of TMJ

These rare lesions may be benign (osteoma, osteoblastoma, osteochondroma, chondromatosis (joint mice)); malignant, from joint tissues (osteosarcoma, chondrosarcoma) or invading from outside the capsule (squamous carcinoma from middle ear or parotid). More rarely, metastatic tumour (breast or prostate) may occupy the condyle head. Diagnosis of any neoplastic change in the TMJ is difficult. While tomography and CT scan help, and Tru-cut needle biopsy is occasionally contributory, it is usually necessary to proceed to direct surgical exploration of the joint to provide adequate tissue for diagnosis. Frozen sections are not always unequivocal; osteoblastoma (benign) is most commonly misdiagnosed as osteosarcoma; the difference is crucial to patient and surgeon!

CLASSIFICATION OF CHRONIC TMJ PROBLEMS

(1) Painful
- (i) Chronic pain dysfunction
- (ii) Disc displacement without reduction
- (iii) Disc perforation
- (iv) Degenerative joint disease (arthrosis, rheumatoid)

(2) Non-painful
- (i) Clicking joint
- (ii) Habitual or long standing dislocation
- (iii) Ankylosis
- (iv) Congenital and developmental disorders

Chronic Pain Dysfunction

The borderland between acute, subacute and chronic pain dysfunction of TMJ is only of academic significance. When the symptoms fail to respond to conservative treatment of suitable duration with modalities such as drugs, physical therapy, occlusal appliances and behavioural modification, yet radiological evidence of degenerative joint disease is absent, the condition is considered intractable and deserving of a fresh approach to management. Revision of the problem should include more sophisticated radiological views, with special emphasis on the diagnosis of discal disorders with and without reduction, and the possibility of perforation of the disc. Double contrast arthrography provides the best opportunity for detection of these chronic intra-articular soft tissue phenomena.

Numerous interventional techniques have been described for the chronically painful TMJ. Occasional intra-articular injection (1–1.5 ml) of steroid suspension (Depo-Medrone, Kenacort A) into the upper joint space alone (relatively simple) or both joint spaces (difficult) may provide long intervals of pain relief. Prior to introducing steroids into the joint a small amount of local anaesthetic should be placed in the preauricular tissues over the condyle neck. Following injection, fullness develops in the ear and joint, tooth contact is disturbed, and the joint should be treated gently for 48 hours. The injection can be repeated 2 or 3 times in a year without risk of iatrogenic steroid necrosis of the condyle.

If the response to intra-articular steroids is disappointing, empirical surgical procedures, such as condylotomy or eminectomy may be attempted. Both operations increase the joint space, either superiorly or anteriorly and reduce the loading of the articular surfaces. High condylar shave achieves a similar immediate result but may lead to inadequate articular repair with painful osteophyte formation. Closed condylotomy with the Gigli saw, once popular, is no longer indicated. A direct approach to the medial side of the condyle neck from a sagittal split-type incision provides direct vision and the additional advantage which accrues to eminectomy and high condylectomy of severing many of the sensory nerve fibres to the painful capsule and synovial apparatus. This operation provides a prolonged period of joint analgesia throughout the recovery period of 2–3 months.

Disc Displacement and Perforation

Where the disc is shown to be folded and fixed in the anterior joint space, open surgical exposure of the disc, reduction into the correct anatomical relationship and plication with sutures to the lateral capsular tissues, is occasionally necessary. Many techniques for disc repositioning have been described; time alone will indicate whether these procedures are more or less successful than condylotomy and high condylectomy, both of which have an excellent record over 30 years.

A perforated disc may be patched with autogenous cartilage (aural) or fascia, lyophilised cartilage, or removed and replaced by a silastic sheet or teflon-lined proplast implant. While it is likely that irregularities in the shape, position or integrity of the disc predispose to degenerative changes in the condyle, the hypothesis cannot be supported by more than presumption. Menisectomy, once popular for the relief of chronic pain dysfunction, was abandoned because of poor long-term results. It is hoped that intra-articular operations to reposition or reconstitute the disc will produce better long-term results.

Degenerative Joint Disease

The onset of pain towards the end of the day, with earache, crepitus and inability to chew, restricted to one joint only, developing gradually in the middle-aged patient (often female) is pathognomonic of degenerative joint disease or arthrosis. Pain may exist, intermittently, for weeks or months before radiological signs of subarticular erosions and microcysts appear. Articular collapse usually follows quickly with gross break-up of the articular cortex over antero-superior aspects of the condylar head. Sugary crepitus and pain are severe.

Given adequate counselling, non-steroidal analgesics (NSAIDs), physical therapy and occlusal adjustment if needed, the condition settles to chronic, diminishing discomfort. Grating in the ear continues long after pain disappears. The condition is spontaneously terminated by repair of the damaged but grossly diminished condylar head. In a small proportion of cases pain and crepitus are intolerable; when response is poor, intra-articular steroids (Kenacort A) at 2–3 monthly intervals, in both joint spaces, may provide analgesia and function. If all these measures fail, condylotomy, high condylar shave or even condylectomy may be required.

Rheumatoid disease

Generally affects the TMJ in about 50% of the afflicted, usually bilaterally. Latex fixation and antinuclear tests may be positive, confirming the diagnosis. Treatment of TMJ rheumatoid disease is best done in conjunction with the rheumatologist. Systemic steroids and gold compounds are reserved for non-responders to less aggressive physical therapy and NSAIDs. Rare complications of long standing TMJ rheumatoid degeneration are necrosis of the condyles with progressive anterior open bite and ankylosis.

Juvenile rheumatoid disease

Affects children, is a more aggressive chronic erosive synovitis of the TMJ, often leading to severe destruction of the condyles and limitation of opening. The effects on growth of the face can be catastrophic. Reconstruction of the damaged or lost condyles is usually left until the disease process is obviously burned out.

Clicking Joint

The clicking joint has already been referred to as occasionally preceding acute onset pain dysfunction in the TMJ. Many joints click noisily and for many years without other symptoms developing. Recent understanding of the normal relationship between the condyle and the disc throughout all stages of the opening and closing cycle has proposed a logical explanation of clicking sounds. The disc can snap or click over the head of the condyle, with the anterior and posterior thickened bands providing a sticking point when hypermobility of the disc is present. Slight hesitancy in disc movement is followed by a return of the disc to its normal relationship with the condyle as elastic fibres in the retrodiscal zone help retraction of the anteriorly dislocated disc.

This phenomenon is now called anterior dislocation of the disc with reduction; clicking sounds may be early or late or both, depending on the stage of the opening or closing cycle at which they become audible. The usual clicking joint responds well to graduated jaw exercises designed to prevent protrusion of the jaw during the early opening phase of mandibular movement. These 'anti-clicking' exercises (see Appendix E., p. 202) done regularly for 3–4 weeks, usually abolish most clicking sounds. When clicking fails to respond completely, sclerosing the lateral capsular ligaments with 0.5 ml STD solution usually produces the final disappearance of unwanted joint noises.

Habitual or Long Standing Dislocation

Habitual dislocation has already been described under acute problems. Rarely, cases are observed where bilateral dislocation, without reduction, has obviously been present for weeks or months. It may occur after general anaesthesia and, occasionally, be not observed postoperatively. The fibrosis associated with the chronic displacement of the joint(s) from the fossa produces a degree of stiffness that prevents simple reduction of dislocation using the local anaesthetic technique described previously.

The addition of a sedation technique using intravenous benzodiazepine to provide muscle relaxation and freedom from anxiety may, in conjunction with adequate local anaesthesia around the joints, permit manual reduction. Usually, however, general anaesthesia with muscle relaxation is used, together with local anaesthetic infiltration; cases of more than 3 months' duration have responded to manual reduction under these operating conditions. If this method fails, small holes can be placed in the angle of the mandible on each side, under general anaesthesia, and traction used to distract the mandible down from the skull. After a short interval, again with the assistance of local anaesthesia, manual reduction can be achieved. Open surgical reduction of the dislocated condyle is not easy to achieve and is not recommended unless the method is employed to reposition a fractured dislocated condyle prior to direct wiring.

Following reduction of dislocated intact condyles it is not necessary to immobilise the jaws. Recurrence of dislocation does not appear to be a problem in cases of reduced long standing dislocation.

Ankylosis

True ankylosis is inability to open the mouth because of changes within the joint proper. Pseudoankylosis is a condition, beyond the capsule of the joint, which affects mobility by mechanical interference.

Causes of true ankylosis

Trauma and infection are both implicated in the onset of ankylosis, particularly in childhood. With the advent of antibiotic therapy, trauma, especially intracapsular fracture of the condyle in childhood, has become the principal cause. In both adult and child a blow transmitted through the long axis of the jaw to the condyle-skull junction may occasionally split the condyle into detached lateral and medial cortical plates which ride up laterally over the outer rim of the fossa and medially into the lateral pterygoid muscle. These fragments unite with the central condylar portion still attached to the neck and bond the condyle to the base of the skull. More rare causes of intracapsular ankylosis are ankylosing spondylitis, Still's disease and advanced rheumatoid arthritis.

Pseudoankylosis

Is principally caused by obstruction to free movement of the coronoid process, either by impaction against an infractured zygomatic arch or because of rare coronoid hyperplasia. Ankylosis of any kind, during active growth, has a profound effect on the downward and forward development of the face and jaws. Relative inactivity of the soft tissues on the affected side(s) fails to provide the stimulus required for growth. Only by early detection and relief of ankylosis can functional development be restored.

Extracapsular ankylosis may be caused by periarticular fibrosis from burns or scars, chronic pericapsular infection (from middle ear or parotid), or long standing dislocation.

Diagnosis of ankylosis

This is occasionally difficult; when there is no detectable movement of either joint it must be established whether ankylosis is unilateral or bilateral. Identification of the affected side, in unilateral cases, is not always clear and unequivocal. Radiographic techniques of tomography and CT scan may be necessary to establish the position and extent of the obstruction to joint movement.

Treatment of ankylosis

Aims of treatment

The aims of treatment are:

(1) To establish joint movement and jaw function
(2) To prevent relapse
(3) To restore appearance and occlusion
(4) To enable unrestricted diet and regular oral hygiene and dental care

Operative techniques are many and varied: all require expert anaesthetic collaboration, with blind intubation or, occasionally, elective tracheostomy. In the child, surgical exposure of the ankylosed area is followed by osteoarthrectomy. When the jaw is freely mobile, the excised condyle is replaced by a costochondral strut from the 8th or 9th ribs, placed to permit adequate restoration of posterior facial height. The procedure may need to be carried out bilaterally.

The surgical approach is usually both preauricular and submandibular when a costochondral strut is secured to the angle of the ramus by osteosynthesis. Postoperative orthodontic supervision is essential and further surgical procedures to improve the appearance may be needed when deformity is severe.

The optimum time for operation in a child with ankylosis is when there is unequivocal clinical and radiological evidence of the condition. When the child is 8–10 years of age, when orthodontic cooperation can be expected, is the ideal time.

In the adult with unilateral ankylosis, osteoarthrectomy from a preauricular approach is followed by interpositional arthroplasty using a pedicled temporal muscle flap anterior to and beneath the zygomatic arch. In cases of bilateral ankylosis, after gap osteoarthrectomy, prefabricated silastic allografts, designed to cover the condylar stump and restore facial height, are secured in position. Active jaw movement commencing 7 days after surgery, whenever possible, should be instituted in all cases after treatment of ankylosis. Intermaxillary fixation is not employed.

Occasionally, in ankylosis of long standing, the coronoid process on the affected side becomes hyperplastic; removal of the hyperplastic tip of the coronoid may be needed at operation to ensure unrestricted movement of the mandible on the mobilised side.

For some time following relief of ankylosis attention should be given to the rehabilitation of the dentition and the removal of interfering dental contacts.

Congenital and Developmental Disorders of the TMJ

Condylar hypoplasia

The condyle and glenoid fossa may be abnormal in a number of craniofacial syndromes. In mandibulofacial dysostosis both condyles are hypoplastic from birth, although the growth and development of the mandible is not obviously impaired by this anomalous form. In the thalidomide syndrome both condyle and fossa are hypoplastic and abnormally placed. Craniofacial microsomia may include hypoplasia or agenesis of the mandibular condyle, unilaterally in about 70% of cases, bilaterally in the remainder. When involvement is bilateral it is not symmetrical. A rare form of symmetrical bilateral agenesis of the condyles has been described.

When the condyle is absent or severely deformed, as part of a craniofacial syndrome, replacement of the articular element of the ramus is usually included in overall surgical reconstruction. Where muscle activity on the affected side offers prospects for growth, early reconstruction of the condylar defect is favoured. Occasionally, in severe damage, costochondral replacement of the condyle is deferred until most active growth is completed. Surgical and orthodontic collaboration are essential in obtaining optimum results from reconstruction of craniofacial deformity of the TMJ.

Condylisis

The term condylisis is used to describe the postnatal loss of a normal condyle. Infection or ischaemic necrosis may be the cause, but the evidence is not always clear. In circumstances where the condyle resorbs but the functional muscle environment remains relatively unaffected, early replacement of the missing condyle by a costochondral graft produces excellent results.

Condylar hyperplasia

A rare form of congenital enlargement of the condyle, ramus and body of the mandible (usually unilaterally) is known as congenital hemihypertrophy. As overgrowth of the affected parts continues until the end of the adolescent growth spurt, surgical (usually cosmetic) reshaping of the mandible is often deferred until all facial growth is completed.

Much more common is developmental hyperplasia of one

mandibular condyle. About the time of puberty, the ramus on the affected side begins to grow asymmetrically. The anterior border of the ramus begins to bow outwards, the condylar neck lengthens and either lateral open bite on the affected side, or crossbite with a swing away from the hyperplastic side, develops. As soon as the signs of this abnormal growth are recognised, collaboration with an orthodontist is recommended. Treatment is most effective when condylectomy, with excision of the condyle head through the neck of the condyle, is carried out before the bite deviation becomes severe. Following condylectomy, remedial exercises may be used to encourage normal jaw function. Orthodontic supervision may be needed to correct any minor irregularities in the occlusion. Excision of the condyle arrests hyperplastic growth. Within one year the condyle head has reformed, but ceases to grow abnormally. No adequate explanation has been provided for the sudden change in growth of the affected condyle.

SURGICAL APPROACHES TO THE TMJ

(1) *Extraoral*—Blind Gigli saw procedure for closed condylotomy. Preauricular approach (with temporal extension for better access anteriorly and superiorly) for condylectomy (high and low), open condylotomy, menisectomy and disc replacement, plication of the capsule, eminectomy, open reduction of condylar fractures, relief of ankylosis.
(2) *Endaural approach*—Seldom favoured except for eminectomy.
(3) *Postauricular approach*—For procedures listed under preauricular approach. Has some cosmetic advantages but may induce stenosis of cartilaginous auditory canal.
(4) *Bitemporal flap approach*—Useful in conjunction with major surgical reconstruction of condyle and zygomatic arch in craniofacial reconstructive surgery.
(5) *Intraoral*—Sagittal split surgical approach for condylectomy, especially of the anteriorly displaced condyle, and for the preferred new medial side open condylotomy procedure.

Note All extraoral approaches to the TMJ may carry some degree of risk to branches of the seventh cranial nerve. All patients undergoing TMJ surgery should be warned of possible facial paresis postoperatively.

Chapter 14

Disorders of the Salivary Glands

There are three major salivary glands, which are paired and situated bilaterally. Minor salivary glands are present in almost every part of the mouth except the gingivae and anterior region of the hard palate. Pathology arising in minor salivary glands may give rise to diagnostic difficulties if their presence and distribution is overlooked.

PAROTID GLAND

The parotid gland is the largest of the salivary glands, is serous secreting, and surrounded by fascia of varying thickness. Superiorly, it is bound by the zygoma, posteriorly, the external auditory meatus, mastoid process and sternomastoid muscle. Inferiorly, it extends into the pterygomandibular space. The accessory gland lies on the main excretory duct which travels over the masseter, pierces the buccinator to emerge opposite the upper second molar. The facial nerve (CN VII) is closely associated with the parotid gland, almost immediately after it emerges through the stylomastoid foramen. The trunk gives rise to its two main divisions which in turn subdivide into at least five main branches.

(1) *Blood supply*

Arterial—Branches of external carotid

Venous—Retromandibular vein

(2) *Lymph drainage*—to glands both within the substance of the parotid as well as superficial to its fascia; then via jugulodigastric and other glands to the deep cervical chain.

Points of Clinical Significance

(1) Learn to examine a preauricular lump, giving precise anatomical landmarks; note extension of the lump into the deep lobe if present. Always examine, therefore, both intra- as well as extraorally.

(2) The close association of the facial nerve means that invasion by a tumour may produce a lower motor neurone palsy. This is an

important sign. The facial nerve is at risk during parotid surgery, especially parotidectomy; patients should be warned.
(3) Learn to locate the parotid papilla for examination, palpation and sialography.
(4) Request a nerve stimulator in cases of parotidectomy. Check whether frozen sections are required, and if so alert the pathology laboratory the day before operation.

Frey's Syndrome

Gustatory sweating (varying degrees of sweating and flushing) of the preauricular skin, is found in approximately one-quarter of patients following surgical removal of the parotid gland. This may occur up to 2 years postoperatively. A starch-iodide test will confirm the phenomenon.

Chronic Parotid Swellings in Children

Unilateral enlargement of the parotid gland is most likely to be caused by a non-epithelial tumour. Approximately 50% of these tumours will be lipomas, angiomas, lymphangiomas or neurofibromas.

SUBMANDIBULAR GLAND

This is the second largest salivary gland and is contained within the submandibular triangle. The deep portion extends below the mylohyoid muscle and extends anteriorly to the anterior belly of the digastric. Posteriorly it curves around the free edge of the mylohyoid muscle to give rise to the deep portion. Laterally it is bound by the mandible. The principal excretory duct (Wharton's) emerges from the deep portion and passes forwards and upwards towards the floor of the mouth.

At first this duct lies on the hyoglossus muscle under cover of the mylohyoid, with the lingual nerve above it and the hypoglossal nerve below. Next it passes to the genioglossus, where the sublingual gland separates it from the mylohyoid and the lingual nerve twists round it, crossing it superficially from above downwards at the anterior border of the hyoglossus and then passing deep to it. The duct runs forward from lateral to medial to emerge adjacent to the lingual frenum.

(1) *Blood supply*
Arterial—Mainly via facial and lingual arteries
Venous—Drains into common facial vein
(2) *Lymph drainage*—From submandibular nodes to deep cervical nodes.

Points of Clinical Significance

(1) Examination of the submandibular gland requires palpation from behind the patient, comparing both sides, and bimanual palpation, from the front. The superficial part of the duct can be easily palpated (e.g. for calculi) using this technique.
(2) Enlarged submandibular lymph nodes may be confused with the gland.
(3) Cannulation of the submandibular duct may be difficult, because of its small size and position. Ask the patient to put the tip of his tongue to the anterior hard palate and then slip the cannula in. A squirt of lemon juice may help stimulate salivary flow from the orifice and hence help location.
(4) Generally speaking, calculi within the anterior part of the duct can be approached surgically through the mouth, whereas symptomatic calculi within the gland substance necessitates gland excision.
(5) The mandibular branch of the facial nerve is at risk during submandibular gland excision. Patients should be warned of this risk preoperatively.

SUBLINGUAL GLAND

This is the smallest of the major salivary glands, situated in the middle region of the sublingual sulcus. Superiorly it is related to the sublingual mucosa and inferiorly rests on the mylohyoid. It is mainly mucous secreting. Its duct (Bartholin's duct) may fuse with the submandibular to produce a common orifice.
(1) *Blood supply*—Lingual artery and branches of the submental artery. Venous return is by corresponding veins.
(2) *Lymph drainage*—Via submental and submandibular glands and hence to the deep cervical chain.

Points of Clinical Interest

A ranula of the floor of the mouth is based on the sublingual gland which must be excised when the ranula is treated or recurrence is likely.

HISTORY AND CLINICAL EXAMINATION

The most common history of salivary gland disease includes:
Swelling
Pain ± swelling
Mouth dryness (xerostomia)
Excessive salivation (sialorrhoea)
Taste abnormalities (usually 'bad' taste)

Swelling

Includes tumours, cysts, mucoceles, sialosis and chronic sialo-adenitis.

Pain and Swelling

Consider:
(1) Acute sialoadenitis—bacterial or viral.
(2) Duct obstruction—swelling and pain associated with eating.
(3) Advanced tumours may well present with nerve paresis and pain.
(4) Drug induced (excessive intake of iodide, lead or mercury) or drug reaction, e.g. phenylbutazone.

Xerostomia

Learn to distinguish between local causes, such as mouth breathing, and serious systemic disease, e.g. Sjögren's syndrome. Factors producing xerostomia may be considered under five headings:
(1) Alteration in fluid and electrolyte balance (often dehydration).
(2) Organic disease of the glands.
(3) Factors affecting salivary centre (rare).
(4) Factors affecting autonomic outflow pathway (often atropine-like agents).
(5) Radiation may predispose the patient to a mucositis as well as xerostomia; excellent oral hygiene should be maintained to avoid rampant caries.

Excessive Salivation

Relatively uncommon. Consider this as either:
(1) Factors affecting higher CNS pathway or salivary centre directly.

(2) Local factors stimulating salivary secretion by reflex, e.g. painful ulcers etc.
It is also commonly seen in various psychiatric disorders.

Taste Abnormalities

Although a bad taste may arise from infected salivary glands, it more commonly arises from infected conditions of the supporting structures of teeth, caries or oesophageal reflux. Taste abnormalities are frequently associated with psychiatric conditions.

USEFUL INVESTIGATIONS

Make a particular note of the duration of symptoms, whether there are any factors which initiate or relieve pain, and with a detailed history and careful physical examination you are in a position to think about further investigations. These are best discussed with your registrar or consultant before initiating further investigations and treatment.

Radiographs

Plain radiographs are particularly useful for demonstrating radio-opaque calculi.
(1) Anterior mandibular occlusal—For calculi in the anterior portion of submandibular duct.
(2) Lateral oblique film of mandible or OPG may show calculi within the substance of the submandibular gland.
(3) A 'soft' PA film may show calculi in the parotid gland or its duct. If intraoral palpation reveals a stone near the orifice, use a small dental film held by the patient over the duct orifice to demonstrate the calculus.

Sialography

Shows the duct and acini by introducing radio-opaque contrast medium. Useful information may be obtained in the diagnosis of calculi (particularly in radiolucent stones), duct strictures, chronic inflammatory conditions, fistulae and neoplastic disease. It is contraindicated where a history of iodine sensitivity is obtained (as contrast medium is often iodine based) or in acute sialoadenitis.

This is a useful technique to learn, and time spent with a radiologist learning interpretation of the sialogram is time invested.

Ultrasound

This non-invasive technique gives useful information on the size, anatomical position and consistency of parotid lumps.

CT Scan

May give further information about the detail of salivary pathology, particularly tumours. Combined sialography and CT scanning occasionally is worthwhile. Discuss this with the radiologist before ordering.

Bacteriology

Pus swabs taken from the duct orifices after massaging the infected salivary gland should be taken before commencing antibiotic therapy. The organism and its antibiotic sensitivity is, therefore, obtained.

Biopsy

Occasionally a percutaneous biopsy of a salivary lump is carried out. A Tru-cut needle or aspiration biopsy are two such methods. These are not techniques to be carried out by the inexperienced. The usefulness of the technique is limited by the reliability of the pathological interpretation. A labial gland biopsy of a minor salivary gland, is however, a much simpler technique and usually involves infiltration of 1 ml of lignocaine with adrenaline into the labial mucosa of the lower lip. A minor salivary gland is located submucosally and submitted for histological examination.

Duct Dilatation

Occasionally orifice or duct stricture gives rise to obstructive symptoms. A lacrimal probe (graded sizes) may be used diagnostically or therapeutically. If you have none in the department try the ophthalmic department.

In the differential diagnosis of parotid problems, it is useful to have a quick check list of what you are likely to encounter. Here is one such breakdown of common methods of clinical presentations.

CHECK LIST

Acute Swellings

(1) Acute sialoadenitis (bacterial).
(2) Viral parotitis—Mumps (myxovirus), Coxsackie A virus etc.

Recurrent Swelling

(1) Punctate sialectasis.
(2) Papillary obstruction—Ulcerative or fibrotic.
(3) Duct obstruction—Within the lumen (e.g. calculi) within the duct wall, and causes outside the wall.
(4) Gland distension—Allergies and drugs.

Persistent Swellings

(1) Benign
Pleomorphic adenoma
Adenolymphoma (Warthin's tumour)
Adenoma (rare)
Oxyphilic adenoma (rare)
(2) Malignant
Pleomorphic adenoma 60%
Adenocystic carcinoma 15%
Adenocarcinoma 10%
Mucoepidermoid carcinoma 10%
Squamous cell carcinoma 5%
Acinar cell carcinoma (rare)

SJÖGREN'S SYNDROME

This comprises a triad consisting of:
(1) Keratoconjunctivitis
(2) Xerostomia
(3) Connective tissue disorders (including 50% that have rheumatoid arthritis)

Middle-aged women predominate in this syndrome and may present with recurrent swelling of salivary or lacrimal glands, together with increasing dryness of the mouth and eyes.

Keratoconjunctivitis is easily recognised: sore, itchy eyes, and decreased lacrimal secretion as shown by testing with filter paper (Schirmer test). Keratitis may be shown by rose bengal staining.

All structures with exocrine glands may be affected, with the production of rhinitis, laryngitis, bronchitis, gastritis and possibly pancreatitis and vaginitis sicca. The dry mouth unaccompanied by swelling of the salivary glands is difficult to assess, as sialographic appearances are non-specific and measurement of salivary secretions difficult and unsatisfactory.

Investigations

Labial gland biopsy is the most useful test, being sensitive, specific and easy to carry out. In the early stage of disease, the histological appearances are non-specific; serological markers of associated autoimmune disease are often present. The combination of a positive rheumatoid factor test, keratoconjunctivitis, and dry mouth is diagnostic in a patient without inflammatory polyarthritis. Antinuclear antibodies, with normal concentrations of DNA antibodies, are frequently present, as are thyroid autoantibodies. The ESR may be raised to 40 + mm/hr.

Treatment

The eye and vaginal symptoms are alleviated by replacement lubricants. Hypomellose eye-drops are generally available and must be used often enough to prevent drying of the conjunctival sac. The dry mouth may be treated with various mouthwashes, saliva substitutes or lozenges. Oral hygiene and topical fluorides must be maintained to prevent progressive caries and periodontal deterioration.

Sicca Syndrome

This consists of keratoconjunctivitis and xerostomia without the associated autoimmune disease.

TRAUMA AFFECTING SALIVARY GLANDS

Trauma to minor salivary glands may produce mucous extravasation or retention cysts, commonly seen on the lips and buccal mucosa, presenting as painless, smooth swellings. Treatment is often surgical excision, and recurrence may be a problem. Alternatively they may be treated by the cryoprobe.

Lacerations to the face and neck may well cut through salivary tissue and a temporary salivary fistula may result. This problem usually settles uneventfully following skin closure and a temporary pressure dressing. If main salivary ducts are cut a sialocele may develop which may be accompanied by a salivary fistula. A sialogram may well be helpful in locating duct transection and duct anastomosis may be required.

Chapter 15

Cranial Nerve Lesions

This chapter is concerned with afflictions of the Vth, VIIth and other relevant cranial nerves. It is based on clinical features and is meant to be a practical guide concentrating on the applied anatomy and most frequent complaints.

FACIAL MOVEMENT (VIIth Cranial Nerve)

Facial weakness (paresis) may arise centrally or peripherally, or be due to primary muscle disease, e.g. myasthenia.

Remember that this nerve has a small sensory component (external auditory meatal and proprioceptive) and that taste and secretory fibres are included within the main trunk in certain sections (see Figure 15.1).

Each half of the upper face is supplied from *both* cerebral hemispheres. Thus when a unilateral lesion occurs above the mid-brain, e.g. stroke, upper facial movement is preserved because of its bilateral cerebral innervation. The lower face, however, being innervated only from the opposite cerebral hemisphere, may well show lower hemifacial paresis.

A lower motor neurone lesion (below the pons) affects functions peripheral to the lesion. If the main nerve trunk is affected, there will be hemifacial paresis, e.g. due to stab wounds, parotid or external jaw surgery, or neoplasia.

Examination

(1) *Movement*—Observe the symmetry and power of facial movement when the patient is asked to show the teeth, purse the lips, 'screw up' the eyes, and wrinkle the forehead.
(2) *Taste*—Sweet, sour, salt and bitter (not commonly tested).
(3) *Secretomotor*—Compare resting with stimulated maximal salivary output (total or parotid) (not commonly tested).

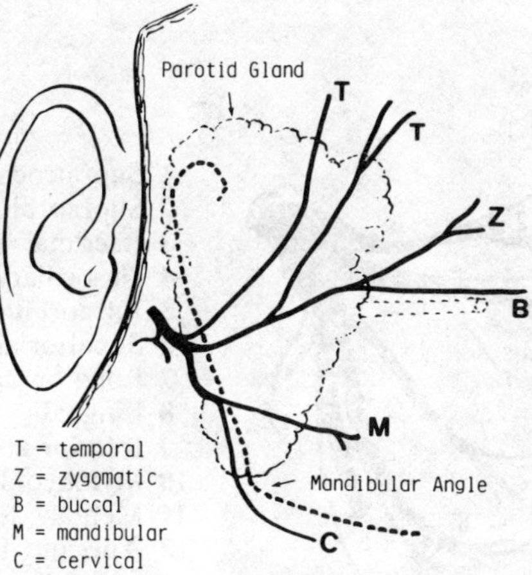

Fig. 15.1 Facial nerve and its branches.

Management

(1) Carry out a general and full neurological examination, looking especially for signs in adjacent cranial nerves V, VI, and VII.
(2) Exclude middle ear diseases/surgery—Test hearing with a tuning fork (Rinne/Weber test that assesses air versus bone conduction, and lateralised acoustic pathology).

Other Causes of Lower Motor Neurone Facial Paralysis

These include head injuries, e.g. fractured skull base, Bell's palsy and diseases in the cerebellopontine angle, e.g. acoustic neuroma.

FACIAL SENSORY DISTURBANCE (Vth Cranial Nerve)

The trigeminal nerve has three trunks, the ophthalmic, the maxillary and the mandibular trunks, and the mandibular branch also carries the motor nerve supply to the masticatory muscles. All the peripheral sensory nerves have their cell bodies in the Gasserian ganglion (see Fig. 15.2, p. 146).

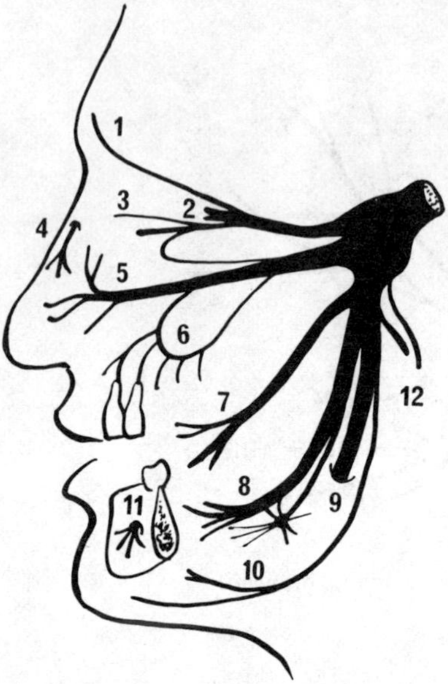

1 Supratrochlear
2 Supraorbital
3 Lacrimal
4 Nasociliary
5 Infraorbital
6 Superior alveolar
7 Long buccal
8 Lingual
9 Inferior alveolar
10 Mylohyoid
11 Mental
12 Auriculo–temporal

Fig. 15.2 Branches of the trigeminal nerve.

Patient History

See Chapter 12 on facial pain.

Examination

Subjective alteration may differ from objective findings.
(1) Test the suspected area for light touch—This involves using a cotton wool point on several areas within the same peripheral nerve distribution. A sterile pin or probe may also be used.
(2) Temperature, vibration and two point discrimination sense—These should be tested.
(3) Motor function—Palpate masseter and temporalis (clenching) and test protrusive movement (lateral pterygoid).
(4) Jaw jerk reflex—With the patient's mouth half open, tap the chin sharply downwards with a patella hammer. A brisk closing response should ensue.

(5) The corneal reflex—Touch the peripheral cornea with cotton wool. This should result in a bilateral blink.

Management of Facial Sensory Disturbance

(1) Exclude oral causes.
(2) Full general clinical and neurological assessment.
(3) Radiographs—Consider taking occipitomental, panoral, intra-oral, submentovertex, lateral and posteroanterior skull and facial bones.
(4) Take a full blood count, check plasma viscosity, blood sugar, Venereal Disease Reference Laboratory (VDRL).
(5) Consider expert neurological referral and ensure long term follow-up to assess any change.

Peripheral Causes of Facial Sensory Disturbances

Surgical treatment

This is performed mainly on the posterior mandibular teeth, careless flap retraction, local anaesthetic injections, endodontic or osteotomy procedures.

Infection

These can be apical infections of lower posterior teeth, upper canines and lateral incisors.

Acute maxillary sinusitis
Infected cysts
Osteomyelitis

Fractures

A blow to a nerve foramen may impair sensation only of the extraosseous portion whereas fractures more commonly compromise the intrabony trunk.

(1) *Inferior alveolar nerve*, e.g. fracture of mandible between the lingula/mental foramen.
(2) *Infraorbital nerve*, e.g. zygomatic, Le Fort II fractures, and orbital floor blowout.
(3) *Anterior ethmoidal nerve*, e.g. nasal fractures, medial wall orbital fractures.

Neoplasm

Infiltration by a malignant tumour can produce progressive sensory impairment, e.g. neoplasm of:

(1) Maxillary sinus, giving infraorbital numbness.

(2) Nasopharyngeal tumours may present with facial sensory disturbance, but other cranial base foramina may also be affected, e.g. IXth and Xth cranial nerve.

(3) Histologically benign tumours within the confines of a bony canal may produce pressure on sensory nerves and impair function, e.g. neuroma.

(4) Any metastatic deposit along the course of a nerve.

Central Causes of Trigeminal Lesions

(1) *Trauma*—Neurosurgical operations or injections.

(2) *Vascular*—Loss of blood supply from certain posterior cranial fossa vessels can result in facial sensory loss in conjunction with other gross long tract signs, such as ataxia.

(3) *Infection*—Particularly of the dural sheaths of the trigeminal roots, e.g. meningitis, petrositis.

(4) *Neoplasm*—Any tumour affecting the cerebellopontine angle can produce facial sensory disturbance.

(5) *Neuropathy*—Multiple sclerosis (disc pallor on fundoscopy), carcinomatous neuropathy; benign trigeminal sensory neuropathy which often affects the cheek (cause uncertain, favours adults, no other clinical signs, non-progressive) syringobulbia.

(6) *Drugs*

(7) *Hysteria*—Usually a younger patient, often female; the disturbance is not commensurate with clinical signs.

CRANIAL NERVE EXAMINATION

I	Smell	If you are uncertain of the patient or his response to the question 'Can you smell normally?', then test. Important causes include injuries to the central mid-third of the face.
II	Sight	Present in each eye? How clear is the sight? Grade visual loss as detecting light, counting fingers, reading large print, or normal size print. This is important in orbital/middle third injuries and surgery to those regions. What are

		the pupil responses to light and accommodation, direct and consensual (beware drug effects).
III IV VI	Binocular eye movements	Ask the patient to focus on your finger at a distance of 1 m and holding his head still ask him to follow your finger. Slowly move your finger to each corner of a square, the centre of which is the visual path direct ahead. Consider charting of movements by orthoptist. Always check this for a patient with orbital injuries awaiting surgery, including patients with zygomatic fractures who have persistent diplopia.
V	Facial sensation	See last section. In addition, is intraoral sensation normal?
VII	Facial movement	See first section.
VIII	Hearing and balance	Is hearing unimpaired on both sides for high and low pitched sounds. Use a 256 Hz tuning fork held to each ear and each mastoid process to confirm that on each side, air conduction is better than bone conduction. Can the patient detect a wrist watch ticking when held close to the ear? Is the patient's balance disturbed? How and in what direction? Possible causes include cranial base fractures, and otitis media.
IX X	Gag reflex	Can gagging be triggered bilaterally? Is soft palatal movement symmetrical? Any suspicion of dysphagia or dysarthria, e.g. Eagle's syndrome, cranial base lesions, neck surgery?
XI	Shoulder injury	Is the bulk of the sternomastoid/trapezius muscles symmetrical? Get patient to hunch the shoulders up towards the ears. Are movements symmetrical, and the shoulders equally strong, e.g. shoulder injuries, radical neck dissection?
XII	Tongue movement	Symmetrical bulk and movement, e.g. protrusion. Is there any evidence of fibrillation or fasciculation ('bags of worms movements'), causes include neck surgery, infiltration by neoplasm, and neurological diseases.

Chapter 16

The Maxillary Antrum

ANATOMY

The maxillary antrum is pyramidal in shape and lined by 'respiratory' epithelium.

(1) The base—Forms part of the lateral wall of the nose.

(2) The apex—Projects laterally into the zygomatic process of the maxilla.

(3) The roof—A thin orbital plate, separating it from the orbit. Running along the roof is the infraorbital canal, containing the nerve, which exits anteriorly into the cheek.

(4) The floor—the alveolar process of the maxilla carries the premolar and molar teeth.

(5) The posterior wall—Separates the sinus from the infratemporal and pterygopalatine fossae. It is pierced by the posterior alveolar nerves which travel to the molar teeth.

(6) The anterior wall—This is the facial surface of the maxilla.

(7) Lymphatic drainage—This is to the submandibular and retropharyngeal nodes. The apices of the 87654|45678 are adjacent to, or intrude into the maxillary sinus. When teeth are lost, alveolar bone is resorbed and the floor of the sinus becomes increasingly thin.

USEFUL X-RAYS

(1) Extraoral—Occipitomental (15° or 45°), lateral skull, orthopantomogram.

(2) Intraoral—Maxillary occlusal, rotated occlusal and periapical films.

(3) Tomography—Plain or CT scans.

Points

(1) Occipitomental views—Probably the most helpful.

(2) Intraoral X-rays—Helpful in defining related alveolar pathol-

ogy. Particularly useful in locating an upwardly displaced tooth or root fragment and in differentiating whether it is extramucosal or within the antral cavity.
(3) Tomography and CT scans—Usually carried out after plain films, if further information is required, e.g. if attempting to define the extent of invasion of a tumour.

ACUTE MAXILLARY SINUSITIS

Acute maxillary sinusitis is usually secondary to an upper respiratory tract infection. It can arise from periapical infection of premolar and molar teeth, or following extractions. The causative organisms include streptococci, staphylococci or anaerobic bacteria. Inflammation of mucosal lining leads to obstruction of ostia.

Symptoms and Signs

(1) Throbbing pain, made worse by head movements or stooping, which may give 'toothache' in premolar or molar teeth.
(2) Tenderness may be elicited over the antrum.
(3) Nasal obstruction may be present.
(4) Mucopurulent discharge may be present under the middle turbinate.
(5) Pyrexia is often present.
(6) The antrum fails to transilluminate. X-rays may show opacity of the sinus and sometimes a fluid level.

Treatment

(1) Antibiotics, e.g. amoxycillin, co-trimoxazole, doxycycline.
(2) Nasal decongestants, e.g. ephedrine nose drops, followed by nasal inhalations.
(3) Analgesics if required.

CHRONIC MAXILLARY SINUSITIS

Signs and Symptoms

These are low grade pain and tenderness, postnasal drip, and halitosis. Chronic infection leads to mucosal hypertrophy and polyp formation. This leads to obstruction of the ostia, which further exacerbates chronic infection. X-rays show opacity or a thickened lining.

Treatment

May consist of one or more of the following:
(1) Antral puncture and lavage. Pus swab obtained for culture and sensitivity (prescribe relevant antibiotic).
(2) Intranasal antrostomy, followed by lavage.
(3) Caldwell-Luc operation. This allows inspection and removal of polyps etc.

Cheek Swelling

(1) Cheek swelling is rare in maxillary sinusitis.
(2) Infected swelling of the cheek is commonly of dental origin, if no skin lesion is apparent.
(3) Swelling of the cheek as a result of antral pathology usually implies malignant disease.

Malignant Disease Within the Sinus

This is uncommon. Approximately 80% of tumours are squamous cell carcinomas. Presentation is often late, hence the poor overall prognosis.

Symptoms and signs

(1) May be no early symptoms.
(2) Blood-stained nasal discharge and nasal obstruction.
(3) Pain or paraesthesia—In distribution of maxillary division of trigeminal nerve.
(4) Eye signs—Proptosis, epiphora and diplopia.
(5) Intraoral signs—Pain or displacement of maxillary teeth, alveolar swelling and delayed socket healing.
(6) Nasal signs—Nasal obstruction, discharge or epistaxis.

Management

(1) Investigation—Plain X-rays, tomography ± CT scans.
(2) Definitive diagnosis—By biopsy, through nose or Caldwell-Luc exploration.

Treatment

This depends on many factors, including evidence of local invasion, metastases, and general health of patient.

A combined radiotherapy/surgical opinion is best obtained to formulate a treatment plan.

RADIOLOGICAL AND CLINICAL FEATURES OF BENIGN LESIONS AFFECTING THE MAXILLARY SINUS

(1) *Osteoma*—Asymptomatic and often an incidental radio-opaque finding which may prevent normal sinus drainage. Gardner's syndrome may present as an antral osteoma.
(2) *Antrolith*—Calcific bodies lying within the sinus which may require removal if they cause symptoms.
(3) *Mucosal cyst (polyp)*—Usually asymptomatic, incidental X-ray findings. A smooth-outlined swelling, often seen on OPGs. These only require treatment if the diagnosis is in doubt or if symptomatic.

Other Cystic Lesions Encroaching on the Sinus

(1) Odontogenic cysts
 Apical, lateral or residual
 Dentigerous
 Keratocysts
(2) Non-odontogenic cysts
Remember that fissural cysts (e.g. nasopalatine, globulomaxillary) may invade the antrum.

Fibrous Dysplasia

Fibrous dysplasia may be monostotic or polyostotic. X-rays show a dense 'ground glass' appearance. It is often asymptomatic.

Presentation

(1) Facial asymmetry, exophthalmos, proptosis.
(2) Continued growth during the period of skeletal growth, then often slows down or stops.

Biopsy

The object of this is to provide a histological diagnosis.

Treatment

Recontour bone.

Paget's Disease

This shows a classic 'cotton-wool' appearance on X-ray. There are difficulties with extractions, delayed healing, liability to low grade infection and propensity for malignant change.

MANAGEMENT OF TEETH IN THE MAXILLARY ANTRUM

Immediate management depends upon the skill of the operator and the facilities available. Firstly, obtain an X-ray to show the position of the tooth fragment. If the fragment is extramucosal, the socket should be judiciously enlarged, and using a small excavator or sucker nozzle an attempt should be made to gently remove the fragment. If this is accomplished, close the socket primarily. Prescribe antibiotics and nasal inhalations.

If the attempt is unsuccessful, prescribe antibiotics and analgesics and seek assistance. This will usually entail removal of the fragment under general anaesthesia. If the fragment of the root is long-standing in the antrum and is completely asymptomatic, both clinically and radiographically, immediate surgical interference is unnecessary. However, clinical or radiological signs of antral infection, the presence of a persisting oroantral fistula or antrolith formation in association with a retained root, gives support to a decision to remove it.

CLOSURE OF OROANTRAL FISTULA

(1) Immediate—If possible carry out primary closure. Prescribe antibiotics and nasal decongestants and advise the patient not to blow his nose.
(2) Late—Spontaneous closure often occurs. If fistula persists review management.

Technique

Operate under local anaesthesia if operator experience and patient tolerance is adequate, otherwise under general anaesthesia.

(1) Raise a generous buccal mucoperiosteal flap.
(2) Incise the periosteum only, to allow tissue advancement over the socket.
(3) Excise the fistulous track in late cases, prior to closure.
(4) Suture flap securely over sound bone. Leave sutures for 7–10 days.

Chapter 17

Common Disorders of the Oral Mucosa

THE ORAL MUCOSA IN HEALTH AND DISEASE

Normal Histology of the Oral Mucosa

(1) Differences from skin
Lack of stratum lucidum—Red colour
No skin appendages such as hair, sweat glands or sebaceous glands (except ectopic ones)
Minor salivary glands
(2) Types of oral mucosa
Masticatory—Keratinised
Lining—Non-keratinised
Special (tongue)—Lingual papillae/taste buds
(3) Normal maturation of the oral mucosa—Reticular, papillary layers of lamina propria, basal layer, stratum spinosum, parakeratotic layer.

Normal Anatomy That May Be Mistaken for Disease

Fordyce spots
Lingual papillae—Filiform, fungiform, circumvallate, foliate
Fissured tongue
Lingual varicosities
Lingual thyroid
Lingual tonsils

Definition of Clinical and Histopathological Terms

Ulcer	total breach of an epithelial surface
Erosion	partial breach of an epithelial surface
Papule	a small raised lesion
Plaque	a slightly elevated lesion with a flat surface
Macule	a reddish brown lesion
Vesicle/bulla	a fluid filled lesion
Pustule	a pus filled lesion

Acanthosis	increase in thickness of the prickle cell (stratum spinosum) layer of stratified squamous epithelium
Acantholysis	loss of adhesion between prickle cells
Hyperkeratosis	increase in thickness of keratin layer
Epithelial dysplasia	abnormal cellular proliferation of epithelium suggestive of changes of a malignant nature (various grades)

Congenital Lesions of Oral Mucosa

White sponge naevus and other congenital keratotic dermatological lesions
Hereditary telangiectasia and other vascular naevi
Hereditary gingival fibromatosis

Traumatic Lesions of the Oral Mucosa

These are all non-specific.
(1) *Mechanical*—Acute, lip, tongue or cheek biting; chronic, occlusal or denture trauma; frictional keratosis from rough restorations or appliances.
(2) *Chemical*—Aspirin burns, caustic agents, cytotoxic drugs all acute; chronic, submucous fibrosis associated with betel nut, slaked lime, etc.
(3) *Physical*—Acute, burns from hot food, drink; smoker's keratosis, cold injury from dry ice cubes, electrical burns from live plugs in mouth; chronic injury from galvanic action of dissimilar restorations; radiation mucositis.
Many factors may combine to produce unusual lesions, e.g. pregnancy epulis associated with trauma and hormonal changes.

Infective Lesions of the Oral Mucosa

(1) *Bacterial infections*—Specific: acute lesions of necrotising ulcerative gingivitis (Vincent's infection) and scarlet fever. Chronic lesions in tuberculosis, syphilis, gonorrhoea (stomatitis and pharyngitis).
(2) *Fungal infections*
(i) Candidosis: acute thrush (hypertrophic) or atrophic form. Chronic, hypertrophic candidal 'leukoplakia'; atrophic form in

denture sore mouth, angular cheilitis. Also associated with multiple hormonal or immunological deficiencies (AIDS).

(ii) Actinomycosis

(iii) Histoplasmosis

(3) *Viral infections*

(i) May involve oral mucosa only; herpes simplex, herpes zoster, herpangina

(ii) Mouth involved as part of a general disease; measles, chicken pox, smallpox, foot and mouth disease, infectious mononucleosis (anginose form), AIDS (HTLV III) infection.

(iii) Chronic viral infections; the viral wart (verruca vulgaris)

(4) *Parasitic infections*—cysticercosis (tapeworm), hydatid cysts

Allergic Diseases of Oral Mucosa

These may be immediate, mainly due to circulating antibodies (steroid treatment) or delayed, mainly due to cell bound antibodies (antihistamine treatment). Penicillin, for example, may produce an acute allergic response (anaphylactic reaction) or generalised drug eruptions. Angioneurotic oedema of lips, pharynx and larynx may be an acute form of drug reaction. Localised contact allergies may arise after restorations containing metals, e.g. nickel, chromium. Skin patch tests may help identify suspected allergies to dental materials. Allergy to local anaesthetics is exceedingly rare; if suspected, refer to allergist for investigation.

Idiopathic Inflammatory Lesions of Oral Mucosa

(1) Geographic tongue

(2) Central papillary atrophy (median rhomboid glossitis)

(3) Recurrent oral ulcerations

Aphthous ulcerations (Mikulicz's ulcers)

Herpetiform ulcers

Periadenitis mucosa necrotica recurrens, PMNR, (major aphthae)

(4) Malignant granuloma (lethal midline granuloma)

Oral Manifestations of Systemic Disorders

(1) *Haematological*

(i) Anaemias

(ii) Leukaemias

(iii) Haemorrhagic disorders
Platelet defects
Vascular wall defects
Coagulation defects
(iv) Leukopenias
(2) *Dermatological*
(i) Maculopapular eruptions
Lichen planus
Lupus erythematosus, psoriasis
(ii) Vesicular (bullous) lesions
Pemphigus
Pemphigoid
(iii) Mucocutaneous ocular syndromes
Erythema multiforme
Behçet's syndrome
Reiter's syndrome
(3) *Nutritional*
Vitamin B group deficiency
Vitamin C deficiency
(Vitamin A deficiency)
Malabsorption syndromes
(4) *Endocrinal*
Postmenopausal syndrome
(5) *Renal disorders*
Uraemic stomatitis
(6) *Reticuloendothelial system*
Lymphomas

THE DIFFERENTIAL DIAGNOSIS OF ORAL MUCOSAL DISEASE

As in all diagnostic exercises, adhere to a step-by-step procedure:
(1) Complete history
(2) Thorough examination
(3) Order special investigations where appropriate

Special Investigations (see also Chapter 5)

(1) Biopsy/cytology
(2) Microbiology

Direct smear
Swab for culture (aerobic, anaerobic, special, e.g. *Candida albicans*, or viruses)
Sensitivity test

(3) Haematology
Screen II—Serum chemistry
Screen III—Complete blood picture
Vitamin B_{12} and serum folic acid
Serum iron

(4) Serology (for syphilis)

(5) Photography

THE DIFFERENTIAL DIAGNOSIS OF WHITE LESIONS IN THE MOUTH

(1) *Developmental*
Oral epithelial naevi (white sponge naevus)

(2) *Inflammatory*
(i) *Traumatic*
Acute—Burns (thermal, chemical, electrical, radiation)
Chronic—Frictional keratosis, smoker's keratosis, cheek biting, lip biting, tongue biting
(ii) *Infective*
Acute—AUG, acute hypertrophic candidosis
Chronic—Mucous patches of secondary syphilis, syphilitic glossitis
(iii) *Idiopathic*
Geographic tongue, idiopathic keratosis, leukoedema

(3) *Neoplastic*
'Leukoplakia' (meaning white patches that cannot be characterised clinically or histologically as any other disease)
Submucous fibrosis
Early squamous cell carcinoma
Some chronic erosive lichenoid lesions

(4) *Oral Manifestations of Systemic Disease*
(i) *Dermatological*
Verruca vulgaris
Lichen planus
Some lesions of discoid lupus erythematosus, psoriasis
(ii) *Haematological*
Plummer-Vinson syndrome

(iii) *Drug-induced*
Butazolidin, Indocid

Treatment of White Lesions

This varies with definitive diagnosis established on clinical grounds, cytology, biopsy, etc.

Leukoplakia is successfully treated by excision with or without skin graft, cryosurgery, laser or topical bleomycin solution. Recurrences should be regarded with suspicion and treated aggressively.

Lichen planus is often resistant to most topical agents including mild antiseptics, steroid ointment, steroid pellets. Erosive lesions may be improved by twice-daily topical steroid sprays. Many white lesions may be reviewed regularly, sometimes with a nuclear stain dye test (toluidine blue or Lugol's iodine) to monitor changes, before being subjected to surgical treatment. Red patches appearing in white lesions increase suspicion of malignant predisposition.

THE DIFFERENTIAL DIAGNOSIS OF ORAL ULCERATION

(1) *Developmental*
Epidermolysis bullosa

(2) *Inflammatory*

(i) Traumatic
Mechanical—Toothbrush trauma, lip/cheek biting
Chemical—Aspirin burn, other caustic burns
Physical—Thermal burns, electrical burns, radiation burns

(ii) Infective
Bacterial—Streptococcal/staphylococcal, gingivo-stomatitis, AUG/Noma, TB, syphilis
Viral—Herpes simplex (primary and recurrent), herpes zoster, herpangina, oral manifestations of systemic viral infections, e.g. measles, chicken pox, infective mononucleosis, foot and mouth disease.
Fungal—Candidiasis (both acute and chronic forms), actinomycosis, other rare fungal diseases such as histoplasmosis
Parasitic—Very rare, such as cysticercosis

(iii) Immunological
Contact stomatitis—Could be due to anything, e.g. dentures, mouthwashes, cosmetics, etc.
Drug allergy—Usually not confined to mouth

(iv) Unknown
Aphthous ulcers, PMNR, herpetiform ulcers, malignant granuloma

(3) *Neoplastic*
(i) Benign lesions are usually not ulcerative unless traumatised
(ii) Malignant ulcers
Primary—'Speckled leukoplakia', 'erythroplakia', carcinoma, others
Metastatic—Most common sites of origin; breast, lung, prostate, thyroid, leukaemia, lymphomas

(4) *Haematological*
(i) Cyclic neutropenia
(ii) Agranulocytosis
Primary
Secondary
(iii) Anaemias
Iron deficiency
Pernicious
Aplastic

(5) *Dermatological*
The mucocutaneous-ocular syndromes
Pemphigus/pemphigoid
Bullous and erosive lichen planus
Lupus erythematosus—Systemic form and discoid form
(Fluorescent autoantibody tests may be needed to confirm diagnosis of pemphigus, pemphigoid, systemic lupus; send frozen biopsy specimen.)

(6) *Endocrinal*
Desquamative gingivitis in postmenopausal females

(7) *Nutritional*
Vitamin B group deficiency

(8) *Urogenital*
Uraemic stomatitis in patients with kidney failure

(9) *Iatrogenic*
Patients receiving cytotoxic drugs, e.g. methotrexate

RECURRENT MUCOUS MEMBRANE ULCERATIONS

Signs, Symptoms, Clinical Features and Treatment

Minor aphthae

Painful ulcers on non-keratinised oral mucous membrane; there are one to five small 5 mm round or oval shallow ulcers, peripheral erythematous halo; recur frequently, often cyclically, heal spontaneously in less than 3 weeks.

Treatment

Bocasan, Difflam, chlorhexidine, carbenoxolone (CBX) mouthwashes, as per preference. Topical corticosteroids occasionally needed. Take care with oral hygiene and acidic irritant foods.

Major aphthae (PMNR)

Painful ulcers on non-keratinised oral mucous membrane; they are large 1–3 cm edged ulcers, and several may be present simultaneously. There is marked tissue destruction sometimes constantly present. Healing is prolonged often with scarring.

Treatment

CBX mouthwash, topical, intralesional, or systemic steroids, cryosurgery occasionally to relieve pain and promote healing.

Herpetiform ulcers

Painful areas of ulceration of keratinised and non-keratinised oral mucous membranes: many small ulcers are clustered together which coalesce forming larger ulcers with irregularly outlined margins. They recur frequently but heal spontaneously in less than 3 weeks.

Treatment

Tetracycline mouthbath, care with oral hygiene and irritant foods.

Behçet's syndrome

Painful ulcers on the oral mucous membranes, conjunctiva or genitalia. Joint lesions or other systemic manifestations may be present. Signs are as for aphthae or herpetiform ulceration; it is usually prolonged.

Treatment

CBX mouthwash, topical or systemic corticosteroids. Take care with oral hygiene and irritant foods. Eliminate possible allergies.

Herpetic ulceration

Multiple ulcers on keratinised and non-keratinised oral mucous membranes, lips and occasionally perioral and perinasal areas. Acute pain. Cluster of vesicles at one site which break down and coalesce forming ulcers with a micropolycyclic margin; marked peripheral erythema. Heal spontaneously in less than 2 weeks; usually appear on lips as 'cold sores'.

Treatment

Symptomatic and preventive; idoxuridine or Acyclovir for lips and CBX mouthbath for intraoral lesions.

Erythema multiforme

Painful ulcers on oral mucosa often with skin, joint, genital or conjunctival lesions; large areas of mucosa involved, covered with fibrinous exudate; blood crusting of lips. Recur infrequently; heal spontaneously in less than 4 weeks.

Treatment

Symptomatic, eliminate allergies especially to drugs. Tetracycline mouthbaths may be of help in idiopathic cases.

Ulcerative lichen planus

Painful ulcers on oral mucosa; skin lesions of lichen planus may also be present; large areas of mucosa may be involved, associated white lesions having a reticular or plaque-like appearance. They are sometimes present constantly and rarely heal spontaneously.

Treatment

Symptomatic and preventive with topical or intralesional corticosteroids.

Benign mucous membrane pemphigoid

Irregular areas of painful ulcerations on the oral mucosa. Bullous skin lesions occasionally present; subepithelial blisters with bleeding occur over large areas of mucosa including conjunctiva, nasal mucosa, pharynx, oesophagus; scarring is a predominant feature, and the Nikolsky sign is positive. They are sometimes constantly present and rarely heal spontaneously.

Treatment

Symptomatic, use topical or systemic corticosteroids. Eliminate oral trauma.

Pemphigus

Ulcers on oral mucosa, often with bullous skin lesions; large blisters often followed by ulceration and bleeding. Nikolsky sign is positive, and progressively increasing areas of mucosa are involved.

Treatment

Symptomatic, use systemic corticosteroids. Eliminate oral trauma.

POTENTIALLY PREMALIGNANT ORAL MUCOSAL LESIONS

Remember the high risk sites: floor of mouth, side of tongue, anterior pillar of fauces.

The risk of malignant transformation is higher in males 45–55 who smoke, drink and neglect dentition. Chronic anaemia and immunocompromised states predispose to malignant change in premalignant lesions.

Suspicious Lesions

Leukoplakia

(1) Period prevalence of malignancy 2.4% in 10 years, 4% in 20 years, i.e. 95% will not become cancer in 20 years.

Speckled or ulcerated leukoplakia is more likely to become malignant. Sublingual keratosis has 50% malignant transformation rate.

(2) Proportion of carcinomas with associated leukoplakia 13–25%. Variation with site and sex; males have more white lesions but in females the malignant transformation rate is higher.

There is a higher incidence of candida in speckled leukoplakia and in leukoplakia becoming malignant. The incidence of candida in cancer is not known.

Nicotine stomatitis

Not usually thought to be premalignant.

Erythroplakia

This is rarer than leukoplakia. There is a higher incidence of epithelial dysplasia. Period prevalence of malignant change and frequency of association with cancer is not proven but suspected to be very high.

Lichen planus

Follow-up suggests 0.5% become malignant
Difficulty of diagnosing lichen planus

Squamous cell papilloma

No data available

Chronic ulceration

No data available

Oral epithelial atrophy

Syphilitic glossitis
Submucous fibrosis
Kelly-Paterson syndrome
Iron and vitamin deficiency

Leukoplakia arising on atrophic epithelium is thought to be more likely to undergo malignant change. However no accurate data exists to confirm this.

Remember 'There is no lethal disease more amenable to effective treatment than oral squamous carcinoma that is less than 1 cm in diameter.'

For treatment of premalignant lesions see Chapter 11.

Chapter 18

Lumps on and Around the Gums (Epulides)

CLASSIFICATION

(1) Firm non-haemorrhagic epulides
(2) Soft haemorrhagic growths/epulides

FIRM NON-HAEMORRHAGIC EPULIDES

Congenital Epulis

(1) It looks like a granular cell myoblastoma.
(2) It is present at birth, located on the gingiva of the maxilla or mandible, more common in the maxilla and is usually pedunculated.

Histology

Large granular cells, similar to a granular cell myoblastoma covered by an atrophic epithelium.

Treatment

Simple excision.

Inflammatory Hyperplasia (Epulis Fissuratum)

This is one of the most common tissue reactions. It is seen as hyperplastic tissue along the denture flange area. Elongated rolls of tissue in the mucolabial or mucobuccal fold are seen. These occur because of denture trauma or resorption of the alveolar ridge.

Histology

Hyperplastic fibrous tissue covered by stratified squamous epithelium with dense collagen, some inflammatory cells and plasma cells.

Treatment

Surgical excision and provision of new dentures.

Squamous Papilloma

This is a common benign tumour of the cheek, gingivae, palate, lips and tongue. It is broad-based or pedunculated with a corrugated or villous surface. Multiple lesions occur in rare syndromes or in association with verruca vulgaris.

Histology

Fronds of squamous epithelium with a connective tissue core.

Treatment

Excision or electrocoagulation.

Fibroepithelial Polyp (Irritation Fibroma)

(1) This is often found in the cheek, tongue, lip and palate.
(2) It is the most common benign lesion occurring in the mouth and can be sessile or pedunculated, firm or soft.
(3) On the gingiva the lesion is often diagnosed clinically as papilloma.

Histology

Dense collagen covered by stratified squamous epithelium.

Treatment

Surgical excision.

Peripheral Fibroma

This is found on the gingiva, is hard and smooth and is a rare lesion of connective tissue covered in stratified squamous epithelium. It may have areas of focal calcification and is then called a peripheral ossifying fibroma.

Treatment

Surgical excision.

Neurofibroma

These arise from cells of the Schwann sheath and fibroblasts. There are two types: numerous, sessile or pedunculated nodules on the skin surface or larger diffuse plexiform lesions. There is an increased incidence of sarcomatous change and lesions can be found intraorally on the buccal mucosa, palate, tongue, gingivae and alveolar ridge.

Histology

Schwann cells with delicate intertwining connective tissue.

Treatment

No satisfactory treatment. These tumours may be removed surgically, but they are rarely solitary.

Lipoma

This is a rare intraoral tumour and can be found on the tongue, floor of the mouth and buccal mucosa. It can be a single or lobulated mass, covered by thin epithelium, yellowish in colour and soft to palpation.

Histology

It is composed of fat cells and has collagen septa.

Treatment

Surgical excision.

Granular Cell Myoblastoma

This is uncommon. The usual site is the tongue and its origin is thought to be either muscle or histiocytes. Lesions in the tongue are usually single nodules within the tongue substance. It can arise on the gingiva, palate and uvula and may be congenital.

Histology

Large granular cells, often intimately related to muscle fibres and nerves, covered by stratified squamous epithelium exhibiting pseudoepitheliomatous hyperplasia which can resemble squamous cell carcinoma.

Treatment

Excision.

SOFT HAEMORRHAGIC EPULIDES

Pyogenic Granuloma

This is a response to a non-specific infection following minor trauma. There is a proliferation of vascular connective tissue which may have rapid growth. Common sites include the gingiva, lips, tongue and buccal mucosa. They may be elevated, sessile or pedunculated. They have a tendency to bleed and are red–purple in colour.

Histology

They are covered by very thin epithelium and have vast numbers of endothelial cells, polymorphs, lymphocytes and plasma cells.

Treatment

Surgical excision.

Pregnancy Tumour

This is histologically identical to a pyogenic granuloma of the gingiva. It occurs during pregnancy, usually in the third month, and increases in size. It usually regresses after pregnancy.

Treatment

Surgical excision is the treatment. However, it may recur if removed during pregnancy as it is a non-capsulated lesion.

Peripheral Giant Cell Granuloma/Epulis

May be due to proliferative response of tissue to injury by tooth extraction, denture irritation or chronic infection. It occurs on the gingiva or alveolar process anterior to the molar teeth and can be either sessile or pedunculated.

Radiographs may show an underlying bony erosion.

Histology

Non-capsulated connective tissue with multinucleated giant cells and numerous capillaries, foci of haemorrhage, and often osteoid and bone is present.

Treatment

Surgical excision and curettage of bone form the treatment.

Brown Tumours

Brown tumours are benign peripheral extensions of intrabony lesions found in hyperparathyroidism. They can resemble giant cell granulomas both clinically and histologically and one must investigate levels of serum calcium, phosphate and alkaline phosphatase.

Chapter 19

Managing the Medical Emergency

CARDIOVASCULAR EMERGENCIES

Collapse

It is important to differentiate between unconsciousness caused by more common conditions (syncope) which respond to simple local measures, and cardiac arrest, which is critical and requires the immediate attention of a trained resuscitation team.

Other Medical Emergencies

These include:

- Faint
- Diabetic coma
- Epileptic fit
- Cerebral haemorrhage

It is possible to differentiate the different types of collapse. If in doubt obtain expert advice immediately.

Syncope

A transient loss of consciousness. Most commonly occurs due to vasovagal attack. Other causes include cerebral arterial disease, low cardiac output, micturition and postural hypotension.

Management

Lie the patient flat, thereby increasing cerebral blood flow. Recovery occurs quickly.

Angina

A clinical diagnosis. Presents as exercise induced retrosternal tightness, often radiates into the neck and down the left arm. Sometimes associated with dyspnoea, nausea and vomiting. Precipitating factors include effort, food, emotion and cold. Relieved by rest and sublingual glyceryl trinitrate. It may be a preinfarction syndrome or crescendo type.

Management

Administer glyceryl trinitrate 0.5 mg sublingually. If no relief within minutes suspect myocardial infarction.

Myocardial Infarction

Myocardial infarction presents with severe crushing retrosternal pain often radiating to the neck and arms of more than 30 min duration; also as acute left ventricular failure and collapse. Patients are often hypotensive, cold, sweaty, anxious, breathless, may have nausea and vomiting and be cyanosed; 25% die suddenly from arrhythmias. A 30–40% mortality occurs in the first 4 weeks, commonly within 48 hours.

Management

(1) Insert an intravenous cannula to aid urgent drug administration.
(2) Analgesia—The following are administered intravenously: diamorphine 5–10 mg or pethidine 50–100 mg plus Maxolon 10 mg (metoclopramide) or Stemetil (prochlorperazine) 12.5 mg.
(3) Oxygen administration—28% (providing the patient is not a carbon dioxide retainer as in chronic obstructive airway disease).
(4) Continuous ECG monitoring.
(5) Arrhythmias are treated as they arise. Bradycardia—By intravenous administration of 0.6–1.2 mg atropine.
(6) If ventricular ectopics or VT (and providing the potassium ion concentration is normal) give lignocaine prophylaxis 100 mg i.v. immediately then commence infusion 2–4 mg/min for 48 hours.
(7) Admit the patient to the intensive care unit, obtain patient history and carry out examination, continual ECG monitoring, chest X-ray, urea and electrolytes, particularly potassium ion concentration, FBC and ESR. Monitor serum cardiac enzymes on three consecutive days (creatinine phosphokinase (CPK) rises within 12 hours) with three serial daily ECGs.

Cardiac Arrest

The patient who has suffered a cardiac arrest has an ashen-grey appearance, and the skin is cold and clammy. In addition the following signs are readily observed:

The patient is unconscious.
There is no pulse in the carotid or femoral artery.
No heart sounds are heard.
The pupils are dilated.
There may be no breath sounds. Monitor to check for ventricular fibrillation, or asystole.

Unless circulation to the brain is restored within 3 minutes, the patient will die or suffer irreversible brain damage.

Management

(1) Summon the arrest team, note time, commence external cardiac message and ventilation.
(2) Lay patient on firm surface. Commence external cardiac massage (ECM) by depressing sternum 4–5 cm at 60/min. Inflate lungs once for every 5 compressions of the chest. Check effectiveness of ECM by feeling for carotid and femoral pulses.
(3) Attach ECG electrodes and monitor the ECG.
(4) Insert an intravenous cannula, run 100 ml of 8.4% sodium bicarbonate rapidly and repeat this with 50 ml every 15 min during the arrest.
(5) Intubate and ventilate with 100% oxygen, 1 inflation per 5 compressions.
(6) *Ventricular fibrillation*—Proceed to DC defibrillation. (If ECG is unobtainable 'blind' defibrillation is justified.) Place the electrode jelly on the defibrillator paddles. Place one electrode to the right of the sternum below the clavicle and the other in the anterior axillary line overlying the 5th left intercostal space. Ensure that nobody else is in contact with the patient at the time of discharge and give 1 × 200 J shock. If there is no result, repeat.

If the second shock fails, double the strength to 400 J and repeat. Between shocks maintain ECM and ventilation. If still in VF, administer 100 mg of lignocaine i.v., maintain the infusion and defibrillate again. If fine ventricular fibrillation persists increase the amplitude by administering 0.5 ml of 1:1000 adrenaline i.v. and repeat DC shock.

If there is still no success, inject phenytoin sodium 100 mg i.v. If successful, continue lignocaine infusion of 2 mg/min for 24–48 hours.

(7) *Asystole*—Indicated by a straight line on the ECG. Administer a sharp blow to the chest. Inject 2 mg of atropine intravenously, 10 ml of 1:10 000 adrenaline, plus 10 ml of 10% calcium gluconate and wait for VF on ECG. When this occurs defibrillate.

If there is no response, repeat adrenaline 10 ml of 1:10 000. If there is still no response inject 5 ml of 1:10 000 intracardiac adrenaline along with 5 ml of 10% calcium gluconate. The needle is inserted to the left of the midline in the 4th intercostal space; maintain the ECM.

Administer 100 ml of 8.4% sodium bicarbonate rapidly, with repeats of 50 ml every 15 min during the arrest.

If resuscitation is successful, admit the patient to the intensive care unit, stabilising with a lignocaine infusion 2–4 mg/min for 24–48 hours, plus dexamethasone 8 mg intravenously 4-hourly for 48 hours to reduce cerebral oedema. If there is evidence of a low cardiac output, commence dopamine infusion of 10 mcg/kg/min.

(8) *Note*—Resuscitation should probably be abandoned if after 30 min there is no evidence of myocardial electrical activity.

(9) After successful resuscitation check for complication of ECM, including fractured ribs and pneumothorax.

Acute Pulmonary Oedema

Acute pulmonary oedema is often found in patients with a previous history of cardiac disease. Usually brought on by left ventricular failure precipitated by myocardial infarct. Presenting signs are acute dyspnoea, pink frothy sputum, cyanosis, sweating, tachycardia, widespread wheezing and crepitations. A chest X-ray shows mottling, Kerley 'B' lines, pleural effusion and often left ventricular enlargement. Asthma, pulmonary embolus and acute or chronic respiratory failure must be excluded. Investigations include a chest X-ray, ECG (look for infarction) and urea and electrolytes.

Management

(1) Sit patient upright, legs dependent and administer 40% oxygen (providing the patient is not a carbon dioxide retainer).

(2) Administer diamorphine 2.5–5 mg i.v. plus Maxolon 10 mg i.v. or Stemetil 12.5 mg i.v.
(3) Give Lasix (frusemide) 40 mg i.v., and monitor potassium level, which may need replacement.
(4) Consider giving aminophylline 250 mg i.v. slowly over 10 min.
(5) Stop all cardiac depressant drugs, e.g. beta-blockers and digitalise only for atrial fibrillation.
(6) Repeat Lasix as required.
(7) If the condition is worsening, positive pressure ventilation may be required. Once the patient is stabilised treat the initiating cause, such as fluid overload, arrhythmias and myocardial infarction. The BP, pulse rate and urine output must be monitored. Check urea and electrolytes twice daily in the early stage.

Deep Venous Thrombosis (see also Chapter 4)

Some patients are predisposed to venous thrombosis in leg and pelvic veins due to venous stagnation, increased clotting tendency and damage to the vascular wall.

Peak incidence is from the second postoperative week and its importance lies in the formation of a pulmonary embolus. High risk patients are the elderly, the immobile, the obese and the postoperative patient.

Signs

Calf tenderness, increased diameter of the calf compared with the other leg, dilatation of superficial veins of the leg and delayed cooling of the leg. Homan's sign is positive. Deep vein thromboses are sometimes symptomless.

Management

(1) Confirm with Doppler flowmetry or venography.
(2) TED stockings are required for clots below the knee; anticoagulate if above the knee.
(3) If proven, anticoagulate immediately with heparin 10 000 units i.v. stat and 1000 units/h, maintaining KCT of 1.5–2.5 times control. After 3 days introduce warfarin checking the prothrombin time. Mobilise after anticoagulation to prevent oedema. Treatment time is 3 months.

(4) ECG/chest X-ray to exclude pulmonary embolus; if this is suspected carry out a lung scan.

Prophylaxis

(1) Early postoperative ambulation, elastic stockings, pneumatic trousers, lower limbs elevated.
(2) *Mini-hep regimen*—Subcutaneous injection of 5000 units calcium heparin 2 hours preoperatively then 12-hourly for 5 days or until ambulation.

Pulmonary Embolism

Occurs when a thrombosis from a deep vein becomes lodged in the pulmonary arterial tree. This usually occurs 10 days postoperatively following bed rest or after myocardial infarction.

(1) *Minor*—Pleuritic pain, haemoptysis, ? shortness of breath.
   Signs—? rub, ± pleural effusion, tachycardia.
   Management—Pain relief with morphine and anticoagulate.

(2) *Major*—Cardiac pain, shortness of breath, ± shock.
   Signs—Raised jugular venous pressure (JVP), fall in blood pressure, tachycardia, gallop rhythm.
   Management—Protect venous return, lie patient flat, relieve pain, avoid diuretics, i.v. fluids till JVP + 8–10 cm of water, 40% oxygen and anticoagulate.

Investigations

Chest X-ray may show a wedge-shaped infarct; ECG is unreliable but it may show S wave in I, Q wave in III and T inversion V 1–4, right axis deviation, right bundle branch block. Lung ventilation perfusion scans should be carried out. Pulmonary arteriography is conclusive.

Administer oxygen because of impaired perfusion and alveolar hypoventilation.

Commence intravenous heparinisation 10 000 units stat, followed by 1000 units/h infusion. Fibrinolytic agents (urokinase or streptokinase) may be preferred but these are rarely used. Embolectomy needed if > 75% of the arterial tree is obliterated on an angiogram.

Hypotensive Crisis

Hypotensive crisis can be caused by a shock syndrome, e.g. hypovolaemic, septic, cardiogenic, anaphylactic and neurogenic shock.

Pathophysiology of Hypovolaemic Shock

Blood loss → Plasma loss → Electrolyte loss

↓

Hypovolaemia
(Activates baroreceptors and sympathetic nervous system)

↓

Arteriolar shutdown

↓

Selective hypoperfusion

↓

Progressive metabolic acidosis

↓

Cerebral acidosis and hypoxia

Signs
Pallor, sweating, coldness, hypotension, tachycardia and air hunger

↓

Assess
Oxygenation—Increase oxygen, maintain airway, hypoxia kills!
Cardiovascular state—Large bore i.v. cannula
Pulmonary state—Blood gases
Renal state—Urinary collection

Fig. 19.1 Hypotensive crisis.

Management

(1) Reverse hypoxia—Administer oxygen 40–60%.
(2) Replace fluids—Initially: colloids—albumin, plasma, Haemaccel, dextran. Later: crystalloids—normal saline. Do not place CVP line in first instance.

(3) Blood gases—Treat acidosis with molar bicarbonate 8.4%, 100 ml of bicarbonate for every 0.1 pH unit.
(4) Ionotropic support if necessary—Dopamine 5 mcg/kg/min.
(5) Renal response—Monitor output, watch for acute renal failure. If there is no urine in 2–3 h use frusemide, mannitol or low dose dopamine (2–3 mcg/kg/min).

Hypotensive crisis affecting organ systems

Cerebral—Mental confusion
Renal—Reduces glomerular filtration
Coronary—Impairs contractility and encourages dysrhythmias

Hypertensive Crisis

This must be treated when a rise in the blood pressure causes left ventricular failure, hypertensive encephalopathy (severe headache, vomiting, confusion, convulsions, visual disturbance) and when the diastolic pressure is greater than 140 mmHg.

Management

Check the blood pressure. If raised this must be treated with care as it is dangerous. Agents used include sodium nitroprusside, hydralazine, diazoxide and ganglion blocking drugs.

Investigations include chest X-ray, ECG, MSU, VMA in urine.

NEUROLOGICAL EMERGENCIES

Coma

A coma is an unarousable lack of awareness attributable to trauma, cerebrovascular accident, metabolic disorder, endocrine disorder, cardiovascular phenomena, epilepsy, infections and intracranial neoplasms.

Friends, relatives, observers and police may provide an instant diagnosis. Obtain a rapid past medical history, examine the patient for evidence of drug abuse, poisons, metabolic upset, e.g. diabetes and hepatic coma, with a careful CNS examination for evidence of cerebrovascular accident (CVA) and meningism.

Plan

Assess the patient clinically, record level of consciousness, pupil reaction and reflexes. Maintain airway and circulation. Initial investigations include full blood count, urea and electrolytes, blood sugar level, drug screen, arterial blood gases, skull and chest radiographs and ECG. Special investigations; skull X-ray and CT scan. Inform the anaesthetist, neurosurgeon or general surgeon of the patient's admission.

Management

(1) Admit the patient to the intensive care unit, to be nursed in semi-prone position.
(2) Check airway, may need intubation and ventilation.
(3) Replace fluid loss by nasogastric tube, i.v. infusion; CVP line if necessary.
(4) Catheterise and commence fluid balance chart.
(5) Maintain caloric intake of at least 1500 calories per day.
(6) Monitor pulse, blood pressure, respiratory rate and neurological observations such as level of consciousness and pupil size and reaction.
(7) Check urea and electrolytes, blood gases and blood glucose. Look for raised intracranial pressure and fitting; check for infection.

General care

(1) Prevent pressure sores by turning the patient 2-hourly, check eye care, oral toilet, physiotherapy, incontinence.
(2) Unconscious patients must be reassessed regularly.
(3) Report a worsening alteration in patient's level of consciousness.

Fitting

Causes include poorly controlled epilepsy, hyperventilation, hypoglycaemia, and lignocaine toxicity.

Treatment

Lie the patient flat, maintain airway, administer oxygen and prevent further injury. The cause of fitting must be investigated.

Status epilepticus

This is where the chronic seizures are longer than 30 min; irreversible cerebral damage can result.
Treatment:
(1) Suppress seizures using diazepam (Valium 10–20 mg i.v. or i.m.) or clonazepam 1 mg i.v., repeat as required. Phenytoin 100–250 mg can also be given by slow intravenous infusion.
(2) Check airway, remove dentures, lie patient in a semi-prone position and administer 100% oxygen.
(3) Check blood levels for anticonvulsant drug, blood sugar level, serum calcium and arterial blood gases.
(4) Commence patient on maintenance therapy and examine for any injuries sustained in the fit.

Delirium Tremens (Acute Alcohol Withdrawal)

This can occur after cessation or reduction of prolonged alcoholic intake resulting in a toxic confusional state and may be fatal.

Symptoms

In the first 2–12 hours of alcohol withdrawal the patient is alert, may have tachycardia and exhibit a slight tremor. After 24–48 hours generalised fits can occur. At 48–96 hours delerium tremens can become manifest by marked agitation, disorientation and hallucinations.

Investigation

Chest X-ray
FBC
Urea and electrolytes
Liver function tests (LFTs)
Blood sugar level (often hypoglycaemic)
Clotting screen

Therapy

(1) Administer chlormethiazole (Heminevrin) *orally* 4–10 g/day in divided doses for 2 days then reduce suggested dose to 3 capsules 6-hourly for 2 days, 2 capsules 6-hourly for 3 days, then 1 capsule

6-hourly for 4 days and stop. Alternatively, i.v. Heminevrin infusion 0.8% (initially 30 ml/10 min) then titrate dose to 0.5–1.0 ml/min to keep the patient sedated.
(2) Take care to avoid respiratory arrest.
(3) In addition Parentrovite 1 ampoule i.m. or i.v. per day prevents Wernicke's encephalopathy, Konakion 10 mg i.m (Vitamin K for clotting).
(4) Monitor progress with FBC, ESR, urea and electrolytes, LFTs, serum folate, vitamin B_{12}, chest X-ray and ECG.
(5) Involve social workers and psychiatrist in the management of these patients.

ENDOCRINE EMERGENCIES

Diabetic Coma

This can be due to either hyperglycaemia or hypoglycaemia. Hypoglycaemia must be excluded in any unconscious patient as irreversible brain damage can occur. Use immediate dipstick to estimate blood sugar level, if less than 2–3 mmol/l (40 mg/100 ml) administer i.v. glucose, 50 ml of 50% dextrose, having first sent off the blood sample for investigation. When in doubt administer glucose. *Never* give insulin as a diagnostic test.

Hypoglycaemia

Rapid onset
Sweating, pale
Rapid full pulse
Low blood sugar level
No glycosuria

Hyperglycaemia

Slow onset
Dry skin, flushed
Dehydrated, hypotensive
Weak, thready pulse
Increased blood sugar level
Glycosuria
Deep sighing respiration because of acidosis, with acetone on breath (Kussmaul's breathing)

Management of hypoglycaemia

(1) Stabilise the blood sugar level by administering 25 g dextrose orally if the patient is conscious, 50 ml of 50% dextrose i.v. or glucagon 1 mg i.m. if unconscious.
(2) Commence i.v. dextrose, monitor blood sugar level with dipstick.
(3) Investigate the cause.

Management of hyperglycaemia

(1) Call physicians
(2) Investigate:
 Packed cell volume (PCV)
 Urea and electrolytes
 Blood sugar level (BSL)
 Check for ketones with Ketostix
 Arterial blood gases
 Blood cultures
 Mid-stream urine specimen (MSU)
(3) Investigate the cause, trauma, surgery, infarction and infection.
(4) Correct fluid loss (rehydrate with normal saline), correct electrolyte abnormalities, acidosis and hyperglycaemia.
(5) Administer insulin at 6 units/h (watch potassium level).

Management of diabetes

Control diabetes by diet, oral hypoglycaemia agents, e.g. sulphonylureas and biguanides or insulin. This may be short-acting or long-acting or combinations of both.

Surgery on the diabetic patient

Discuss the planned surgery with anaesthetist, where possible the patient should be first on list (see Chapter 3).
(1) *Diet control*—Stabilise preoperative and postoperative blood sugar levels, no special precautions.
(2) *Oral hypoglycaemic control*—If good control omit morning dose on operation day and test preoperative and postoperative blood sugar levels. Poor control, stop all drugs. Patients require dextrose insulin drip preoperatively.

(3) *Insulin control*—Admit for preoperative assessment, stabilise blood sugar level and test preoperatively. The patient often requires a dextrose insulin drip (5% dextrose i.v. with 10 units/l soluble insulin) operatively titrated according to blood sugar level. Post-operatively monitor blood sugar level 4-hourly using BM stix or Dextrostix, commencing on normal diet as soon as possible. Arrange a morning operation, no insulin on the operation day. If late morning or afternoon operation, halve normal dose in morning and set up 5% dextrose i.v. infusion per operation.
(4) *Dextrose insulin drip*—Ten units of soluble insulin in 500 ml of 5% dextrose. Run in over 5 hours, i.e. 100 ml/h, monitoring with BM stix.
(5) *Post surgery*—Monitor blood glucose 4-hourly until stable (6–10 mmol/l) and patient is able to eat. In the meantime control with i.v. 5% dextrose and insulin infusion pump.

Blood glucose mmol/l	Soluble insulin
<4	0.5 units/h
4–15	2.0 units/h
>15<20	4.0 units/h

Steroid Crisis (Addisonian Crisis)

The adrenals release endogenous steroids when the body is subjected to stress. Long-term steroids lead to adrenal cortex atrophy. Adrenal failure may occur with failure of the hypothalamic (pituitary) adrenal cortex axis.

An absence of steroid response to stress can result in hypotension, collapse and death. Response is depressed in patients who are on or have received steroids in the past year and are subjected to infection, trauma and surgical stress.

Signs

Apathy, hypotension, vomiting and coma.

Management

(1) Monitor blood pressure half-hourly.
(2) Investigate full blood count, PCV, urea and electrolytes, BSL.
(3) Give 200 mg of hydrocortisone (100 mg i.m., 100 mg i.v.) plus 100 mg i.m. 8-hourly.

(4) Administer intravenous normal saline 1 l in 2 hours then maintain CVP within the normal range.
(5) Monitor urea and electrolyes and BSL and supplement where necessary.
(6) Maintain blood pressure chart and investigate cause of crisis.

Preventing steroid crisis

(1) *Minor surgery*—If no steroids have been administered in the past 18 months no supplement is required. If steroids during this period, give hydrocortisone 200 mg i.m. and continue present regimen.
(2) *Major surgery*—Hydrocortisone 200 mg i.v. preoperatively and 200 mg 6-hourly postoperatively for 48 hours.

RESPIRATORY EMERGENCIES

Asthma

Diagnosis on a history of episodic wheeze and dyspnoea which are recurrent and reversible. Usually initiated by infection, allergy or emotion.

Signs

Dyspnoea, tachycardia, wheeze, use of accessory muscles of respiration.

Management

(1) Assess respiratory function, Peak Expiratory Flow Rate (PEFR), Forced Expiratory Volume (FEV 1) for baseline measurements.
(2) Investigate with chest X-ray, FBC, arterial blood gases, sputum for microscopy, culture and sensitivity (MC & S).
(3) Commence treatment by nebulised salbutamol (Ventolin) using 1 ml of 0.5% salbutamol 4-hourly, plus infusion of 500 mg of aminophylline in 1 litre of normal saline over 24 hours.
(4) Treat hypoxia with 40% oxygen plus. (You cannot give too much oxygen with asthma.) Alternatively i.v. aminophylline 250 mg slowly over 10 min and commence aminophylline infusion. If the attack is severe add 100 mg of hydrocortisone i.v. 6-hourly.

(5) Treat infection with antibiotic of choice, usually Amoxil. Keep the patient hydrated as this decreases sputum stickiness; physiotherapy essential.
(6) Monitor patient's improvement with repeat respiratory function tests and blood gases. The mainstay of treatment is *oxygen*, *bronchodilatation*, *physiotherapy* and *antibiotics*.
(7) Consider ventilation if:
$Pao_2 < 6.5$ kPa
$Paco_2 > 6.5$ kPa
pH < 7.3
Systolic BP < 90 mmHg

Acute Laryngeal Obstruction

The patient experiences distress and forced respiratory effort. Coughing and stridor on inspiration are present, if not corrected cyanosis and unconsciousness occur.

Causes

Inhalation of foreign body, angio-oedema, trauma, infection, facial burns.

Management

(1) Establish airway, inspect pharynx and larynx to remove foreign bodies if present.
(2) If obstruction is due to food bolus, perform 'Heimlich manoeuvre'. Press forcibly with fist below the xiphoid process pushing the diaphragm up and expelling air from mouth, thus clearing airway.
(3) If there is no improvement, carry out emergency cricothyrotomy (see Chapter 6).
(4) In the case of angio-oedema, administer adrenaline 0.5 mg 1:1000 subcutaneous /i.m. with hydrocortisone 200 mg i.v. ± chlorpheniramine (Piriton) 10 mg i.v./i.m.

Pneumothorax

This is a condition where air escapes into the pleural cavity. May be spontaneous (ruptured bulla) or traumatic in origin.

Symptoms

Pleuritic pain, dyspnoea.

Signs

A combination of diminished movement on the affected side, tracheal displacement (unreliable), hyperresonance on percussion, decreased respiratory sounds on affected side. Confirm with chest X-ray.

Management

This involves insertion of an intercostal drain for underwater seal (see Chapter 6).

Mendelson's Syndrome (Inhalation of Vomitus)

Vomiting is a particular hazard during general anaesthesia in the induction and recovery stages. It occurs because intra-abdominal pressure is greater than the competence of the sphincter at the lower end of the oesophagus and material can overspill into the respiratory tract. The normal stomach emptying time is 4–5 hours. Metoclopramide (Maxolon) increases peristalsis and hence speeds emptying time, whereas a fatty meal slows emptying time. Hence the patient must have no food or drink 6 hours before operation, or aspirate stomach contents in the case of an emergency operation.

Management of a patient following inhalation of gastric contents

(1) Suck out contents of the pharynx and larynx.
(2) Mendelson's syndrome is characterised by bronchospasm, circulatory collapse, pulmonary oedema and death in about 25% of cases.
(3) Administer aminophylline 250 mg i.v. slowly.
(4) Administer hydrocortisone 200 mg i.v. stat and repeat 100 mg hydrocortisone 6-hourly for 48 hours.
(5) Ventilate the patient, commence on antibiotics and chest physiotherapy, following the progress clinically and with a chest X-ray.

Respiratory Arrest

Respiratory arrest can be primary or secondary: primary arrest is caused by drug overdose, sedation, hysteria or by airway obstruction with a foreign body; secondary arrest can follow cardiac arrest.

Signs

No respiratory movement and cyanosis.

Management

(1) If drug induced—administer naloxone, doxapram and ventilate.
(2) Clear the airway, inflate lungs using mouth to mouth resuscitation 12 times per minute and if possible ventilate with 100% oxygen; feel for pulse, and if absent external cardiac massage is required.

Signs of respiratory failure needing support

Respiratory rate is >30/min; pH<7.2; $Paco_2$>6.0 kPa; Pao_2<10 kPa (on 40% oxygen).

Hyperventilation Syndrome

Overbreathing can occur with anxiety and hysteria. Alveolar Pco_2 and subsequently the plasma Pco_2 is lowered causing cerebral ischaemia. This results in light headedness, dizziness and also loss of consciousness. Paraesthesia may occur around the mouth and in the arms and legs. Carpopedal spasm may be seen due to relative hypocalcaemia. The patient becomes distressed and a vicious circle is set up.

Treatment

(1) Reassure, have patient breathe in and out of paper bag so $Paco_2$ increases and reverses tetany and breaks the cycle of events.
(2) On recovery demonstrate to patient the precipitating factors.
(3) Hyperventilation may be caused by salicylate overdose—Hence exclude.

DRUG INTERACTIONS

Anaphylactic Shock

This is a severe allergic reaction most commonly attributed to drug atopy, e.g. penicillin sensitivity and can result in death.

Signs

Urticaria, bronchospasm, laryngospasm, hypotension, circulatory collapse with a fall in blood pressure. The skin is pale, sweaty and ashen-grey.

Management

Administer adrenaline 0.5 ml of 1:1000 i.m. or 0.2 ml of 1:1000 adrenaline diluted in 10 ml of normal saline given slowly intravenously. Repeat at 15 minute intervals until there are signs of improvement.
(1) + Chlorpheniramine (Piriton) 10 mg. i.v. slowly or i.m.
(2) ± Hydrocortisone 200 mg i.v. (of secondary value as onset of action is delayed for several hours).
(3) ± Aminophylline 200 mg i.v. slowly over 10 minutes for bronchospasm + 100% oxygen. ? Ventilate if necessary.
First line treatment is restoration of blood pressure, lie patient flat, raise feet, infuse 5% dextrose saline or dextran 70.

Angio-oedema

Angio-oedema results from increased vascular permeability as a result of an allergic reaction. The more common type is due to type I and II hypersensitivity. Patients undergo rapid oedematous swelling around the head and neck and this can be a lone occurrence or be associated with anaphylaxis.

Treatment

Adrenaline, steroids and chlorpheniramine injections. Tracheal intubation may be necessary. Prophylaxis is with Pro-Actidil.

Hereditary angioneurotic oedema (HANE)

This occurs with deficiency or inactivity of C_1 esterase inhibitor, resulting in continual activation of complement-like substances causing an increase in capillary permeability. Confirm the diagnosis by the assay of C_1 esterase inhibitor and C_4.

Signs

Tense non-pitting oedema of the face, neck, hands, feet, genitalia and gastrointestinal tract. Episodes of painless swellings subside in 24–48 hours. There is danger if oedema extends to the glottis. Can be initiated by trauma.

Management

(1) Fresh frozen plasma, i.v. tranexamic acid (antifibrinolytic agent) prior to surgery.
(2) Long term prophylaxis with anabolic steroid Stanazol (raises C_1 esterase inhibitor).

Chapter 20

Record Keeping

One of the house surgeon's most important and onerous duties is to keep good clinical records and correspondence.

WHY DO GOOD RECORDS MATTER SO MUCH?

(1) They facilitate safe, efficient, continuous clinical care.
(2) For medico-legal purposes, as an *aide memoire* for preparing reports and for self-defence if professional conduct or competence should be challenged. Good quality records imply good clinical care and vice versa.
(3) For research.

THE HALLMARK OF GOOD RECORDS

They should be:
(1) Accurate and complete.
(2) Legible.
(3) Relevant *quality* is more important than *quantity*.
(4) Signed and dated.
(5) Contemporary: later alterations should be initialled and dated.
(6) Factual and professional (and contain no obscenity, blasphemy, sarcasm, invective or misplaced humour).
(7) Free from obscure or misleading abbreviations.
The consultant should guide each new house officer on the established practice and procedures of the department, including those relating to record keeping.

HOSPITAL LETTERS AND REFERRALS

The referring practitioner needs to be kept informed of the patient's progress and discharge. General practitioners often complain about lack of information from the hospital, especially if they are being asked to remove sutures, prescribe drugs or follow-up the case.

If there is any delay in despatching the formal hospital discharge summary, an interim note containing the essential points should be sent, perhaps with the patient. But if a patient is used as a postman, it should be anticipated that he/she will open and read the letter.

Referral of an in-patient to another specialist should be arranged personally and courteously through the proper channels and with the provision of sufficient clinical information.

THE PREPARATION OF MEDICO-LEGAL REPORTS

General principles:

(1) Obtain the patient's consent (only *unnecessary* when the report is requested by the patient's own solicitor).

(2) Ascertain the purpose of the report and state this and give the addressee at the beginning.

(3) State the patient's full name, address, date of birth and occupation.

(4) If the author has never seen the patient personally but has prepared the report from the records only he should say so.

(5) If the report is produced after a special examination, give the date, time and place of it.

(6) Summarise the history of the case firstly as given by the patient, and secondly as revealed by any contemporary clinical records or other evidence.

(7) Summarise the findings on examination and the results of special investigations, e.g. X-rays.

(8) Summarise the treatment given to date.

(9) Give an opinion on prognosis, mentioning any permanent disability or the need for and cost of future treatment.

(10) In case of personal injury it may be important to comment on causation, but it may not be possible to say more than 'the findings on examination were *consistent with* the history given'. If you were not present you cannot say how the accident happened.

(11) Keep within the limits of your own knowledge and expertise.

(12) Remember that one day you may be examined and cross-examined in court on your report.

DISCLOSURE OF NOTES FOR LITIGATION PURPOSES

In the UK there is no automatic right for a patient or his lawyer to gain access to clinical records, but a High Court procedure exists to permit, in appropriate circumstances, an *application* for an order for release of *relevant* records. In this sense, records are not as private and confidential as some imagine. The golden rule is only to record what you would be happy to read out in court in public.

The consultant in charge of the case, the hospital administrator and your defence organisation should be consulted and will help if questions of disclosure arise.

CERTIFICATION

Registered dental practitioners are required to exercise great care in issuing certificates and similar documents and should not sign statements which they have not verified. The issue of a false or misleading statement may render the practitioner liable to legal and professional disciplinary proceedings. In short, one should always read and consider carefully the details of any form or certificate before completing and signing it.

HANDOVER OF PATIENTS

Before going 'off duty', the house surgeon must be sure that proper arrangements have been made for the continuing care of his patients. This means communicating adequately with the nursing staff and with the colleague who is to deputise for the house surgeon.

CONSENT AND WARNINGS

Most in-patients will be asked to give informed written consent to operation. It is usually the house surgeon's job to explain the nature and purpose of the proposed procedure. He should use terms which the patient can understand and should countersign the consent form. This is a very responsible task. If the house officer does not understand the operation himself, e.g. in cases of orthognathic surgery or trauma, then he should ask the registrar or consultant to deal with the consent issue.

In every case appropriate warnings of possible complications must be given. In oral surgery the risk of iatrogenic nerve injury is a classic instance. The house officer should ascertain the department's policy from his senior colleagues. Case law shows that the patient must be warned of problems and complications which are genuinely likely to occur. Whatever warnings are given should ideally be recorded in the notes.

SUMMARY

Good clinical notes are a vital part of good clinical practice and will always help both patient and practitioner.

Appendices

A. ERUPTION DATES

Deciduous Teeth

Eruption commences at about 6 months and is completed by $2\frac{1}{2}$ years. The following dates are approximate, mandibular before maxillary.

Table 1
Approximate Eruption Dates for Deciduous Teeth

Teeth	*Time (months)*
Incisors	6–9
Canines	16–18
First molar	12–14
Second molar	20–24

Permanent Teeth

Root formation is complete at 2–3 years posteruption.

Table 2
Approximate Eruption Dates for Permanent Teeth

Teeth	*Time (years)*
Incisors	6–8
Canines	10–12
First premolar	10–11
Second premolar	11
First molar	6
Second molar	12

B. CEPHALOMETRIC TABLES

(mean values)

SNA	81°
SNB	79°
ANB	1–3°

Skeletal Class I ANB = 2–4°
II ANB >4°
III ANB <2°

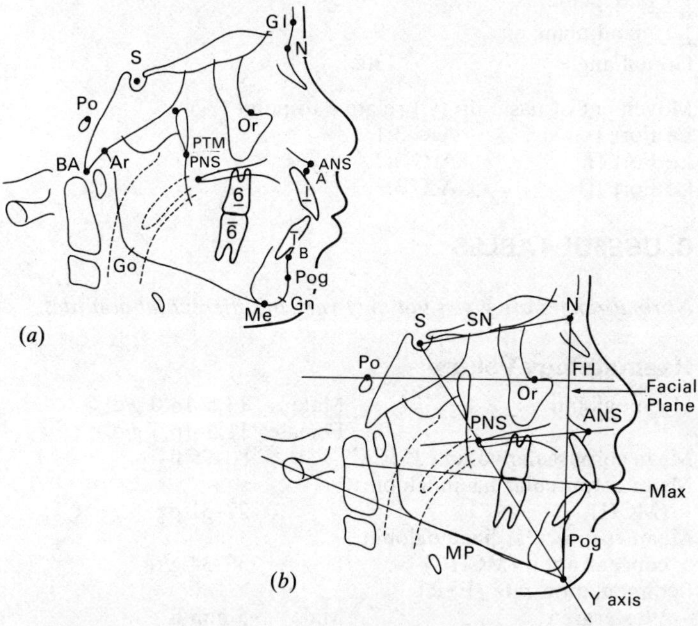

Anterior Nasal Spine (ANS), Articulare (Ar), Basion (BA), Frankfort horizontal (FH), Gnathion (Gn), Gonion (Go), Mandibular plane (MP), Maxillary plane (Max), Menton (Me), Nasion (N), Orbitale (Or), Pogonion (Pog), Point A, Point B, Porion (Po), Posterior Nasal Spine (PNS), Pterygomaxillary fissure (PTM), Sella (S), Sella - Nasion (SN).

Fig. A.1 (*a*) and (*b*) Common cephalometric reference points, lines and planes.

Vertical Facial Height Measurements

ATFH (N–Me)	= 120 mm (all approximate normal values)
AUFH (M–ANS)	= 55 mm
ALFH (ANS–Me)	= 65 mm
PTFH (SN–Go)	= 79 mm
PUFH (SN–PNS)	= 46 mm
PLFH (PNS–MP)	= 43 mm
MMA	25–30°
SN:MP	32°
1/1 max plane	109°
1/1 mand plane	90°
Gonial angle	130°

Movement of nasal tip (C) relative to point (A)

Le Fort I	A:C 3:1
Le Fort II	A:C 3:2
Le Fort III	A:C 3:3

C. USEFUL TABLES

Normal ranges are given but may vary in different laboratories.

Haematology Values

Haemoglobin	Male	13.5–18.0 g/dl
	Female	11.5–16.5 g/dl
Mean corpuscular volume (MCV)		80–96 fl
Mean corpuscular haemoglobin (MCH)		27–31 pg
Mean corpuscular haemoglobin concentration (MCHC)		30–34 g/dl
Sedimentation rate (ESR) Westergren	Male	5 mm/h
	Female	7 mm/h
Platelets		150–400×10^9/l
Packed cell volume (PCV, haematocrit)	Male	42–52% (0.42–0.52)
	Female	37–47% (0.37–0.47)
Erythrocytes	Male	4.6–6.2×10^{12}/l
	Female	4.2–5.4×10^{12}/l
Reticulocytes		0.2–2.0% (25–100×10^9/)

Leucocytes		
Total		$4.0–10.0 \times 10^9/l$
Neutrophils		$2.5–7.5 \times 10^9/l$
Lymphocytes		$1.5–3.5 \times 10^9/l$
Monocytes		$0.2–0.8 \times 10^9/l$
Eosinophils		$0.04–0.44 \times 10^9/l$
Serum ferritin	Male	24–187 ng/ml
	Female	14–130 ng/ml
Serum iron	Male	13–36 μmol/l
	Female	12–31 μmol/l
Total iron binding capacity (TIBC)		44–72 μmol/l
Serum folate		3–20 μg/l
Red cell folate		160–640 μg/l
Serum B_{12}		150–925 ng/l
Bleeding time (Duke's method)		2–7 min
Clotting time (venous blood—glass test tube)		5–11 min
Prothrombin time I, II, VII, X		11–14 s
Activated partial thromboplastin time VII, IX, XI, XII		30–40 s
Prothrombin index = $\frac{\text{control time (s)}}{\text{patient time (s)}} \times 100$		
Bl volume—mean	Male 69 ml/kg	
	Female 65 ml/kg	

Clinical Chemistry

Sodium	137–146 mmol/l
Potassium	3.5–5.0 mmol/l
Calcium	2.1–2.6 mmol/l
Chloride	97–108 mmol/l
Bicarbonate	23–31 mmol/l
Phosphate	0.8–1.5 mmol/l
Urea	3–8 mmol/l
Creatinine	50–130 μmol/l
Uric acid	120–500 μmol/l
Glucose (fasting)	3.0–5.6 mmol/l (56–100 mg/100 ml)
Bilirubin	3–17 μmol/l
Alkaline phosphatase	3–13 King Armstrong units/dl (30–300 IU/l)

Protein	
Total	60–80 g/l
Albumin	35–50 g/l
globulin	15–30 g/l
Fibrinogen	1–5 g/l
Arterial Blood Gases	
pH	7.36–7.42
Pa_{O_2}	80–100 mmHg (10.6–13.2 kPa)
Pa_{CO_2}	34–46 mmHg (4.5–6.0 kPa)
Standard bicarbonate	21–26 mmol/l
Base excess	±2 mmol/l (7.6 mmHg = 1 kPa)
Enzymes	
Acid phosphatase	1–5 IU/l
Alkaline phosphatase	30–300 IU/l
Amylase	<200 somogyi units
Aspartate aminotransaminase (AST)	10–50 IU/l
Creatinine phosphokinase (CPK)	<130 IU/l
Hydroxybutyrate (HBD)	100–250 IU/l
Lactic dehydrogenase (LDH)	90–300 IU/l

Intravenous Fluids

Administered to:
- replace fluid lost
- maintain normal daily requirements

In an emergency use colloids or crystalloids for replacement, later crossmatched blood if necessary
- Colloids—Albumin, dextran, Haemaccel
- Crystalloids—0.9% normal saline, 5% dextrose, dextrose saline

Daily requirements = 3000 ml fluid.

One standard regimen—1 l 5% dextrose, 1 l normal saline, 1 l 5% dextrose over 24 h.

Normal saline 0.9% has same sodium content as plasma (150 mmol/ l).

5% Dextrose contains no sodium, 278 mmol/l glucose (50 g/l), and produces 200 kCal/l energy.

Dextrose saline 30 mmol/l of sodium, 222 mmol/l of glucose.

Blood Transfusion

(1) Check correct crossmatched blood.
(2) Monitor BP, P, temperature and urine output.
(3) Never give less than 2 units blood (1 unit raises Hb by 1–1.5 g/dl).
(4) Transfuse at a rate of:
  1 unit/2 h (unless shocked)
  1 unit/4 h in the elderly

If prone to heart failure give frusemide 40 mg i.m./i.v. with each unit.

Diabetic Patient

Blood glucose 2.5–5.6 mmol/l
Diabetes mellitus random blood glucose level (BGL) >11.0 mmol/l
Place the blood sample in a yellow cap fluoride bottle.
Monitor:
  Urine
  Capillary blood (finger prick) Diastix / BM stix } spot testing

Monitor long-term control by glycosylated haemoglobin

Normal	7% of Hb is glycosylated	
Diabetic patient	7–9%	good control
	10–12%	moderate control
	13–20%	poor control

D. SPECIMEN BOTTLES

Haematology

Full blood count, Red cell indices, Whole blood folate } EDTA tube, gently mix to prevent clotting
Serum ferritin, Serum iron, Total iron binding capacity, Serum B_{12} } Plain tube clotted blood
ESR, Prothrombin time } citrated tube
Blood group and crossmatch—Plain tube
Clotting studies arrange with haematologist
Biochemistry—Blood glucose in fluoride bottle (yellow)
  Urea and electrolytes use lithium heparin (orange)
Immunology—Use serum, plain tube

Microbiology—Pus in sterile container, send to laboratory. If kept longer than 2 h, put swab in transport medium and refrigerate at 4° C.
Viral studies—Swab in viral transport medium, serum in two specimens with a 2 week interval.
Histology—In 10% formal saline.

E. REMEDIAL JAW EXERCISES FOR THE TEMPOROMANDIBULAR JOINT

(1) Exercise for pain/dysfunction syndrome.
*Use vapour coolant spray over affected joint as directed before commencing exercises *or*
*Give both jaw joints preliminary warmth with a protected hot water bottle or infra-red lamp applied to first one joint, and then the other for 10–15 min on each side before commencing exercises.
**Cross out the section which does not apply*

Reflex opening exercise. Partly open mouth against hand pressure on chin for 20–30 seconds; swallow, to relax, then open smoothly and widely without deviation, supporting both jaw joints with light finger pressure.

Lateral opening movement. Support first the left jaw joint with fingers of the left hand and place the right hand against the side of the right jaw; open with a sideways swing to the right against firm pressure from the right hand.

Do the lateral opening exercises on the opposite side.

Do each exercise in turn and repeat the whole series six times, three times a day to begin with, then reducing gradually to two a day, one a day, three times a week, etc. until completely free of pain.

(2) Exercise to prevent clicking of the jaw joint.
The exercise should be carried out sitting in an erect posture in front of a mirror; it should be done at least twice daily in this position until the art of contracting the muscle beneath the chin has been completely mastered.

Clasp both hands behind the nape of the neck to provide a 'headrest'.

With the mouth closed and the teeth lightly touching, contract the muscle beneath the chin, attempting to pull the chin back into the neck without opening the mouth. By observing the chin and neck in the mirror it is possible to see the contractions of these suprahyoid muscles.

For the first few days do not move the jaw or teeth when doing the exercise. *Once the art of muscle contraction is learned* it should be done for 3–5 min of each hour, not necessarily sitting, or in front of a mirror.

With practice a definite sensation of tension will be noted in the suprahyoid muscles and in the region of the jaw joints.

Once the essential exercise has been learned it can be done with small mouth opening movements, learning to open the jaw with a backward pull, and avoiding the 'click'.

Gradually increase the extent of mouth opening until it can be opened to the full normal extent without producing a 'click'—always keep the suprahyoid muscles retracted.

Remember Muscles can be coaxed, but not driven; if this exercise is practised for 2–3 weeks it will become second nature and the click will not return.

F. ASSESSMENT OF LEVEL OF CONSCIOUSNESS USING THE GLASGOW COMA SCALE

Eye opening		
spontaneous	4	E
to speech	3	
to pain	2	
nil	1	
Verbal response		
orientated	5	V
confused conversation	4	
inappropriate words	3	
incomprehensible sounds	2	
nil	1	
Motor response		
obeys	6	M
localises	5	
withdraws (flexion)	4	
abnormal (flexion)	3	
extensor response	2	
nil	1	

Observations are recorded on a chart, 2-hourly, over each 24 hours and a graph drawn. The duration of coma can thus be defined more precisely, as can the extent of recovery in the longer term. Maximum score of E + M + V = 15; minimum = 3.

G. TOLUIDINE BLUE SCREENING METHOD FOR RECOGNITION OF ORAL MALIGNANCY

Prepare toluidine blue stain as follows:

Tolonium chloride powder 1 g
Acetic acid 10 ml
Absolute alcohol 4.19 ml
Distilled water 86 ml

This mixture makes 100 ml of a 1% solution of tolonium, adjusted to pH 4.5 or less.

Technique

(1) Clean surface of area to be tested by swabbing with 2% acetic acid solution.
(2) Dry surface with gauze; apply 1% tolonium solution liberally to surface of mucosa under investigation.
(3) Rinse for several minutes with vigorous mouth washing.
(4) Decolorise tissues by swabbing thoroughly with 2% acetic acid solution again.
(5) Dry tissues and search for accumulations of bright blue dye in tissues. The nuclear stain is concentrated in cells undergoing intense mitotic division.

This technique may be used to detect unobserved, asymptomatic oral mucosal cancers after clinical examination, and for monitoring persistent oral mucosal lesions which are not ulcerated but remain abnormal in appearance. After a positive stain, repeat stain test 10–14 days later. A further positive stain makes biopsy of the lesion mandatory.

Bibliography

Banks P. (1981). Killey's Fractures of the middle-third of the facial skeleton. In: *Dental Practitioner Handbook No. 3*. Bristol: John Wright and Sons.

Banks P. (1983). *Killey's Fractures of the Mandible*. Bristol: John Wright & Sons.

Bell W. E. (1985). *Orofacial Pains: Classification, Diagnosis and Management (3rd edn)*. Chicago: Year Book Medical Publishers Inc.

Fraenkel G. J., Ludbrook J., Hill G. L., Marshall V. R. (1980). *Guide for House Surgeons in the Surgical Unit*. London: William Heinemann Medical Books.

Gilbertson A. A. (1984). *Intravenous Technique and Therapy*. London: William Heinemann Medical Books.

Henderson D., Poswillo D. E. (1985). *A Colour Atlas and Textbook of Orthognathic Surgery*. London: Wolfe Medical Publications.

Henk J. M., Langdon J. D. (1985). *Malignant Tumours of the Oral Cavity*. London: Edward Arnold.

Howe G. L. (1985). *Minor Oral Surgery*. Bristol: John Wright and Sons.

Hughes-Jones N. C. (1979). *Lecture Notes on Haematology*. Oxford: Blackwell Scientific Publications.

Killey H. C., Kay L. W. (1975). *The Maxillary Sinus and its Dental Implications*. Bristol: John Wright and Sons.

Killey H. C., Seward G. R., Kay L. W. (1975). *An Outline of Oral Surgery*. Bristol: John Wright and Sons.

Mason D. K., Chisholm D. M. (1975). *Salivary Glands in Health and Disease*. London: W. B. Saunders and Co. Ltd.

Moore J. R., ed. (1985). *Surgery of the Mouth and Jaws*. Oxford: Blackwell Scientific Publications.

Richards P., Truniger B. (1983). *Understanding Water, Electrolyte and Acid Base Balance*. London: William Heinemann Medical Books.

Robinson R., Stott R. B. (1983). *Medical Emergencies: Diagnosis and Management*. London: William Heinemann Medical Books.

Rowe N. L., Williams J. L. (1985). *Maxillofacial Injuries*. Edinburgh: Churchill Livingstone.

Scully C. (1985). *Hospital Dental Surgeons Guide*. London: British Dental Journal.

Scully C., Cawson R. A. (1982). *Medical Problems in Dentistry*. Bristol: John Wright and Sons.

Shafer W. G., Hine M. K., Levy B. M. (1983). *A Textbook of Oral Pathology*. London: W. B. Saunders and Co. Ltd.

Shear M. (1983). *Cysts of the Oral Regions*. Bristol: John Wright and Sons.

Shklar G. (1984). *Oral Cancer*. London: W. B. Saunders and Co. Ltd.

Smith N. J. D. (1980). *Dental Radiography*. Oxford: Blackwell Scientific Publications.

Stell P. M., Maran A. G. (1978). *Head and Neck Surgery (2nd edn)*. London: William Heinemann Medical Books.

Westaby S. (1985). *Wound Care*. London: William Heinemann Medical Books.

Glossary of Abbreviations

Ab	Antibody
ACTH	Adrenocorticotrophic hormone
ADH	Antidiuretic hormone
Ag	Antigen
AIDS	Acquired immune deficiency syndrome
ANF	Antinuclear factor
ANK	Appointment not kept
APTT	Activated partial thromboplastin time
ARF	Acute renal failure
AS	Aortic stenosis
ASD	Atrial septal defect
AST	Aspartate transaminase
ATS	Antitetanus serum
AUG/ANUG	Acute necrotising ulcerative gingivitis
AV	Arteriovenous
BCG	Vaccine against TB
BGL/BSL	Blood glucose/sugar level
BMMP	Benign mucous membrane pemphigoid
BNF	British National Formulary
BP	Blood pressure
BPC	British Pharmacopoeia
BRA	Bite raising appliance
BSR	British standard ratio (prothrombin index)
BW	Bitewing
Ca	Cancer
CAT/CT scan	Computerised axial tomography
CBC	Complete blood count
CBX	Carbenoxolone (Bioplex mouthwash)
CCF	Congestive cardiac failure
CCU	Coronary care unit
CD	Controlled drug
CDH	Congenital dislocation of the hip

CDO	Chief Dental Officer
CFT	Complement fixation test
CHD	Congenital heart disease
CHF	Congestive heart failure
CI	Contraindications (drugs)
CLP	Cleft lip/palate
CMO	Chief Medical Officer (DHSS)
CMV	Cytomegalovirus
CN	Cranial nerve
CNS	Central nervous system
CO	Complaining of
COAD	Chronic obstructive airways disease
CPC	Clinicopathological conference
CPK	Creatinine phosphokinase
CPR	Cardiopulmonary resuscitation
CRF	Chronic renal failure
CSF	Cerebrospinal fluid
CSSD	Central sterile supplies department
CV	Curriculum vitae
CVA	Cerebrovascular accident
CVP	Central venous pressure
CVS	Cardiovascular system
CXR	Chest X-ray
DDAVP	Desmopressin
DHA	District Health Authority
DIC	Disseminated intravascular coagulation
DIF	Direct immunofluorescence
DLE	Discoid lupus erythematosus
DMT	District medical team
DNA	Did not attend
DPF	Dental Practitioners' Formulary
DS	Disseminated sclerosis
DT	Delirium tremens
DVT	Deep vein thrombosis
DXR	Deep X-ray radiation
EACA	Epsilon aminocaproic acid
EAM	External auditory meatus
EBV	Epstein-Barr virus
ECG	Electrocardiogram

ECM	External cardiac massage
ECT	Electroconvulsive therapy
EDTA	Ethylenediaminetetracetic acid (chelates Ca, Mg, K, Na)
EEG	Electroencephalogram
EM	Electron microscope
EMG	Electromyogram
EMU	Early morning urine
ES	Extra systoles
ESR	Erythrocyte sedimentation rate
FB	Foreign body
FBC/FBP	Full blood count/picture
FDPs	Fibrin degradation products
Fe	Iron
FEV	Forced expiratory volume
FH	Family history
FRC	Forced residual capacity
FTA	Fluorescent treponemal antibodies
GA	General anaesthesia
GIT	Gastrointestinal tract
GM	*Grand mal*
GMH	General medical history
GPI	General paralysis of the insane
GTT	Glucose tolerance test
GU	Genitourinary
Hb	Haemoglobin
HbS	Haemoglobin S (sickle cell)
HBsAg	Hepatitis B surface antigen
HBV	Hepatitis B virus
HDL	High density lipoproteins
HLA	Human leukocyte antigen
HPC	History of present complaint
HPI	History of present illness
HPV	Human papilloma virus
HSV	Herpes simplex virus
HTLV	Human T cell lymphotropic virus
IA	Intra-arterial

IC	Immune complex
ICP	Intracranial pressure
ICU	Intensive care unit
Ig	Immunoglobulin (+IgG, IgA, IgM, IgE)
IHD	Ischaemic heart disease
IIF	Indirect immunofluorescence
IM	Intramuscular
IMF	Intermaxillary fixation
IP	Intraperitoneal
ITU	Intensive treatment unit
IV	Intravenous
IVC	Inferior vena cava
IVP	Intravenous pyelography
IVU	Intravenous urogram
JVP	Jugular venous pressure
KCT	Kaolin cephalin time
LA	Local anaesthesia
LDL	Low density lipoproteins
LE	Lupus erythematosus
LFT	Liver function tests (serum bilirubin and 'liver enzymes', e.g. AST and GGT)
LH	Luteinising hormone
LHF	Left heart failure
LIF	Left iliac fossa
LKKS	Liver, kidneys, spleen
LLSD	Lower labial set down
LMN	Lower motor neurone
LMP	Last menstrual period
LP	Lumbar puncture
LVF	Left ventricular failure
LVH	Left ventricular hypertrophy
MAOI	Monoamine oxidase inhibitors
MCH	Mean corpuscular haemoglobin
MCHC	Mean corpuscular haemoglobin concentration
MC&S	Microscopy, culture and sensitivity
MCV	Mean corpuscular volume

MDU	Medical Defence Union
MEC	Medical Executive Committee
MI	Myocardial infarct
MIMS	Monthly Index of Medical Specialities
Mini-hep	Subcutaneous heparin
MND	Motor neurone disease
MPDS	Mandibular pain dysfunction syndrome
MPS	Medical Protection Society
MRI/NMR	Magnetic resonance imaging
MS	Multiple sclerosis
MSU	Mid-stream urine
NAD	No abnormality detected
NSAID	Non-steroid anti-inflammatory drug
NSU	Non-specific urethritis
NTR	No treatment required
OA	Osteoarthritis
OAF	Oroantral fistula
OM	Occipitomental view
OPT	Orthopantomograph
PA	Perapical or postero-anterior views
$P\text{CO}_2$	Partial pressure of carbon dioxide
PCV	Packed cell volume
PDA	Patent ductus arteriosus
PEFR	Peak expiratory flow rate
PERLA	Pupils equal reacting to light and accommodation
PHT	Pulmonary hypertension
PLS	Persistent lymphadenopathy syndrome
PM	*Petit mal*
PMH	Past medical history
PMNR	Periadenitis mucosa necrotica recurrens (major aphthae)
$P\text{O}_2$	Partial pressure of oxygen
POM	'Prescription only' medicine
PR	Per rectum, or pulse rate
PS	Pulmonary stenosis
PT	Prothrombin time
PTH	Parathyroid hormone
PTTK	Activated partial thromboplastin time

PUO	Pyrexia of unknown origin
PV	Per vaginam
RA	Rheumatoid arthritis, or relative analgesia
RAU	Recurrent aphthous ulceration
RCT	Root canal treatment
RBBB	Right bundle branch block
RF	Rheumatoid factor
RFT	Renal function tests
Rh	Rhesus
RHA	Regional Health Authority
RhF	Rheumatic fever
RHF	Right heart failure
RIF	Right iliac fossa
ROU	Recurrent oral ulceration
RRF	Retrograde root filling
RTA	Road traffic accident
RVF	Right ventricular failure
SA	Subarachnoid
SBE	Subacute bacterial endocarditis
SC	Subcutaneous
SG	Specific gravity
SI	International System of Units
SLE	Systemic lupus erythematosus
SMV	Submentovertex view
SOA	Swelling of ankles
SOB	Shortness of breath
SOL	Space-occupying lesion
SS	Sagittal split osteotomy
STD	Sexually transmitted diseases, or sodium tetradecyl sulphate (sclerosant)
SVC	Superior vena cava
TB	Tuberculosis
TFT	Thyroid function tests
TIBC	Total iron binding capacity
TLC	Tender loving care
TMJ	Temporomandibular joint
TPHA	*Treponema pallidum* haemagglutination test
TPI	*Treponema pallidum* immobilisation test

TPR	Temperature, pulse, respiration
TRH	Thyroid-releasing hormone
TSH	Thyroid-stimulating hormone
TSSU	Theatre sterile supplies unit
TT	Thrombin time
U&E	Urea and electrolytes
UGS	Urogenital system
UMN	Upper motor neurone
URTI	Upper respiratory tract infection
UTI	Urinary tract infection
VC	Vital capacity
VDRL	Venereal Disease Reference Laboratories screen
VF	Ventricular fibrillation
VMA	Vanillylmandelic acid
VSD	Ventricular septal defect
VSS	Vertical subsigmoid osteotomy
VT	Ventricular tachycardia
VV	Varicose veins
WBC	White blood count
WCC	White cell count
WR	Wasserman reaction

Index

Notes